Society and Health in Guyana

Society and Health in Guyana
The Sociology of Health Care in a Developing Nation

Marcel Fredericks
John Lennon
Paul Mundy
and
Janet Fredericks

CAROLINA ACADEMIC PRESS
Durham, North Carolina

© 1986 by Marcel Fredericks, John Lennon, Paul Mundy, and Janet Fredericks
All rights reserved.

Library of Congress Catalog Number: 84–70752
International Standard Book Number: 0–89089–295–4

Carolina Academic Press
Post Office Box 8795, Forest Hills Station
Durham, North Carolina   27707

Design by Anistatia Renard
Printed in the United States of America

To the late Dr. Frederic Gardiner Rose
O.B.E.; B.A.; M.R.C.S. (Eng.); L.R.C.P. (London); M.D.;
B.Ch. (Camb.); D.M.R. and E., (Camb.); M.R.C.P. (London)

Pioneer in the Research of Hansen's Disease
Friend of the poor, the sick, and the forgotten ones
in the Republic of Guyana, South America
May he rest in peace

About The Authors

Dr. Marcel Fredericks was born in Guyana, South America. He is professor in the Department of Sociology-Anthropology, Loyola University of Chicago. Dr. Fredericks obtained his School Certificate with distinction from the University of Cambridge and matriculated from the University of London, England. He received his Ph.D. degree in medical sociology from Loyola University of Chicago. He established the Office of Research in Medical Sociology and has since served as its director. Dr. Fredericks has twice been awarded a United States Public Health Service Fellowship for research and teaching at the Harvard University Medical School and was later appointed research associate in pediatrics there. With Dr. Mundy he has written on medical and dental sociology, including *The Sociology of Health Care, The Making of a Physician, Making It in Med School*, and *Dental Care in Society: The Sociology of Dental Health*. Other books include: *First Steps in Sociology, Citizen Jesuit* and *Hosting of The Foreign Student*.

Dr. John Lennon is professor of sociology, University of Arkansas at Little Rock. He received his A.B. degree from John Carroll University, his M.A. degree from The Catholic University of America and his Ph.D. from the University of Notre Dame. Dr. Lennon has published widely in various scholarly journals. His book *A Study of the Acculturation and Assimilation of Puerto Rican Families in Chicago* has received wide acclaim. His areas of specialization include Urban Sociology, Criminal Justice and Law, Juvenile Delinquency and Social Problems. He is co-author of *First Steps in Sociology*.

Dr. Paul Mundy, professor of sociology, Loyola University of Chicago, received his B.A., *magna cum laude*, from the University of Scranton. He was awarded his Ph.D. with distinction from The Catholic University of America, where he later directed the undergraduate program in sociology. He served for four years with the Princeton University Office of Population Research in international demographic studies. At Loyola he has been primarily responsible for developing its graduate program in sociology and has also served as department chairman. He has been editor of the *American Catholic Sociological Review* and president of the American Catholic Sociological Society and the Religious Research Association. He is co-author of *The Making of a Physician, The Sociology of Health Care, Making It in Med School, Dental Care in Society: The Sociology of Dental Health, First Steps in Sociology,* and *Citizen Jesuit.*

Dr. *Janet Patricia Fredericks,* formerly principal of Notre Dame de Chicago, received her B.S. and M.Ed. degrees from Loyola University of Chicago. Her M.A.L.S. degree was obtained from Rosary College, Graduate School of Library Science, and her Ph.D. was awarded by Loyola University of Chicago. She has recently completed the volume *The Education Views of Lyndon Baines Johnson* and has co-authored *Hosting of The Foreign Student.* She has also presented papers in the Society of Educational Biography. Dr. Fredericks teaches in the Department of Educational Foundations and in the Department of Curriculum and Instruction, Loyola University of Chicago. She is also the educational coordinator of the American Institute of Banking, Chicago, Illinois.

Foreword

The dynamics of progress in a society is a reflection or a product of change. True, all change cannot always be recognized as a social good. Such a conclusion introduces a question of values or an appraisal in terms of a point of reference. Such a reference point may be the status preceding the onset of change, in which case it becomes a baseline, or it may be the planned goal towards which the calculated change is being projected. In any case, development is a function of change.

Guyana is changing; it is developing; it is progressing. As a developing country new to the experience of independence, charting its own course in the rough seas of international diplomacy and commerce, without the sheltering umbrella of a mother country on which it once had so depended, Guyana is experiencing all the pangs of an undeveloped country seeking to develop its own identity. Like other countries in similar circumstances, it has been experiencing the travail of economic survival in a world dominated largely by the hegemony of entrenched capitalism. Capitalism as an economic philosophy is a bulwark for the "haves" and frustration and despair to the "have nots." This is true in a national as well as an international context. Free unrestricted enterprise, in the competition of an open market, brings little cheer and no prospect of gain to those who have little with which to trade. In such a setting, the strong grow stronger; they survive and thrive at the expense of the weak. For the economically deprived, the terms "subsidy" or "charity" must be added as an amendment to the law of supply and demand. The governments of the world's poor countries recognize this, and their reactions are dictated by stern necessity. The first recourse has been in the imposing of controls. In some countries, these can be all-pervasive, involving not only production and distribution but also the exchange and utilization of services. To such governments, economic controls are an inevitable expediency if they are to effectively mobilize the limited resources of their struggling country in order to meet the challenges and needs of a restive and hungry population. In this respect, Guyana perhaps has been more fortunate than many of the other newly independent countries. It has had no sustained experience of violence. True, for a brief period following Independence, there were fears of a civil war; but the calm, firm, even-handed administration of the Burnham government has discouraged overt violence and has persuaded its critics to seek redress in the ballot box.

The government of Guyana is not communistic; it is socialistic. This is not an exercise in semantics. While capitalism in its expression is monolithic, socialism is polytypic. Every country defines, for itself, its concept of socialism. In Guyana, the government describes its ideology as "co-operative socialism," defined as a system in which all the barriers of discrimination in any category are legally abolished and the economic, social, and cultural resources of the country are mobilized and so distributed as to benefit all the citizens.

With the above foreword and background, one can now better appreciate the personal scope of Dr. Marcel Fredericks' sociological contribution on Guyana, for Dr. Fredericks was born in Guyana. The many years that he has lived away from the country have obviously not dulled his love for the place of his birth. Throughout this work, one can sense a nostalgia as he scans the structure and fabric of Guyana as a society. He scans its history as a colonial fief to the many imperial colonizing nations of Europe. He describes the multi-ethnic population in terms of its various origins, customs, folklore, traditions, and contributions to the Guyana society. He addresses himself to the changes, political and economic, to which the society is reacting. His review of the changing health pattern as a consequence of changing attitudes towards hygiene, environmental sanitation, and food value is interesting. He is impressed by Guyana, struggling as it is against discouraging odds to bring to all of its citizens the opportunity to enjoy a better standard of life.

E.L.C. Broomes, B.S.C., M.D., F.I.C.S., A.A, LL.D.
Honorary Consul for the Republic of Guyana

Acknowledgments

Our thanks are extended to all the students whom we have taught at the undergraduate, graduate, and professional levels at the Loyola University Schools of Medicine, Dentistry, Nursing, and Education; the University of Arkansas; and the Harvard University Medical School. We are grateful for their concern, comments, and questions about health care in developed and developing nations. In a sense, they demanded that this book be written.

In a very special way, the authors are most grateful to Dr. Edward L. C. Broomes—Honorary Consul to the Republic of Guyana, physician, surgeon, and a native Guyanese—for his painstaking efforts in reading various typed copies of the manuscript. His editorial contributions to this volume are appreciated. We are also pleased to thank his gracious wife, Mrs. Anna Broomes, for her valued assistance in dealing with foods and beverages. To Ambassador Lawrence Mann and his staff at the Guyana Embassy in Washington, D.C., we are thankful for the most recent information on health care facilities in Guyana. We appreciate the services on this project of Dr. Adegbola Adejunmobi of Nigeria and Sonia Aladjem, as Research Assistants in the Department of Sociology and Anthrolopology.

Here at Loyola, we wish to thank Fr. Raymond C. Baumhart, S.J., President; Dr. Richard Matre, Provost of the Medical Center; Dr. Ronald E. Walker, Senior Vice-President and Dean of Faculties; Dr. Thomas J. Bennett, Director of Research Services; Mr. Edward Powers; and Dr. John Tobin for their interest and valuable assistance in many different areas.

We happily acknowledge our debt to Fr. Lawrence Biondi, S.J., Dean of the College of Arts and Sciences; Dr. Kathleen McCourt, Chairperson of the Department of Sociology and Anthropology; as well as Susan Frissell, Yolande Wersching, Rhodda Thompson, Rev. William Grogan, and Thomas Hitcho for reading the final version of the manuscript.

Our gratitude is extended to Dr. Patricia Rose, physician and surgeon, Department of Public Health, Public Hospital Georgetown, Guyana, for her permission to use the research data on Hansen's disease.

We also wish to acknowledge and give credit to Anthony Fredericks for providing the photographs in this volume. All of the photographs were taken in 1980. Also, to Paul Edward Fredericks, Barrister-at-Law and

Director of Shell Oil Company, we are grateful for permission to utilize the health care data of Dr. George Giglioli, retired medical advisor to the Guyana Sugar Producers' Association.

Finally, Dr. Fredericks wishes to extend his thanks to the late Dr. John Kosa. During his U.S. Postdoctoral Health Service Fellowship years of research and teaching at the Harvard Medical School, he had the opportunity to discuss with Dr. Kosa the many ramifications of health care in Guyana.

Contents

About the Authors	v
Foreword	vii
Acknowledgments	ix
List of Illustrations	xiii

1	Guyana: The Land and Its People	1
	Culture in Guyana	3
	The Political Situation in Guyana	7
	Summary	10
2	Health Services	11
	History of the Georgetown Hospital	11
	Health Care Developments: 1933–1966	12
	Structure of Present-day Health Services	17
	Preventive Medicine	17
	Environmental Sanitation Program	18
	District Hospitals	20
	New Georgetown Hospital	21
	Services for the Hinterland	23
	Geriatric Unit	23
	Community Aid in Health Services Development	23
	The General Development Plan for Guyana's Health Services	24
	Summary	25
3	Public Health Services	27
	Health Services Before Independence	27
	Development and Future of the Malaria Eradication Campaign	28
	Current Public Health Services	37
	Summary	40
4	Health Education in Guyana	43
	History of Education	43
	Current Educational Development	46
	Medical Research Conference	51
	Summary	56
5	Hansen's Disease in Guyana	57
	Early Treatment Ensures Complete Cure	57

xii Contents

6 Physicians in Guyana ... 67
   Characteristics of the Social Background of Guyanese Physicians ... 67
   Factors in the Decision on a Field of Practice ... 68
   Physicians' Attitude Toward the Medical Profession ... 68
   Outstanding Physicians in Guyana ... 70
   Summary ... 77

7 Folk Medicine Practices in Guyana ... 79
   Concern for Proper Health Care ... 82
   Dental Care ... 84
   Summary ... 85

8 Changing Health Care in a Changing Guyana ... 87
   Problems of Families ... 87
   Family and Sick Role ... 88
   Family Typology ... 91
   New Times—New Problems ... 92
   The Sudden Fall of Death and Birth ... 96
   A Tale of Two Countries ... 97
   Summary and Epilogue ... 100

Appendix I: Geography of Guyana ... 101
Appendix II: Brief History of Guyana ... 109
Appendix III: Amerindians Today ... 113
Appendix IV: Constitution of Guyana ... 117
Appendix V: Constituent Assembly ... 119
Appendix VI: Guyana's Cultural Heritage ... 121
Appendix VII: Religious Festivals ... 125
Appendix VIII: National Flag of Guyana ... 127
Appendix IX: 1980 Budget ... 129
Appendix X: Education in Guyana ... 131
Appendix XI: Major Industries in Guyana ... 137
Appendix XII: Local Substitutes for Foods Unavailable in Guyana ... 139
Appendix XIII: Health Facilities in Administrative Districts ... 141
Appendix XIV: Fertility, Mortality, and Morbidity Trends ... 147
Appendix XV: Historical Note ... 151

Notes ... 155
Recommended Readings ... 159
Glossary ... 163
Index ... 171

List of Illustrations

Map of Guyana	xiv–xv

Greater Georgetown (East) Health Center, Campbellville	120
Municipal Day Care Center (Creche)—South Road, Georgetown	108
Public Hospital, Bartica, Essequibo	120
St. Joseph Mercy Hospital, Georgetown	118
Medical Arts Center, Thomas Center, Georgetown	118
Public Hospital, Georgetown. View from Thomas Street	116
David Rose Center, West Ruimveldt	128
Red Cross Convalescent Home for Children, Parade Street, Georgetown	116
Municipal Welfare Center, South Ruimveldt, Greater Georgetown	128
Beterverwagting Triumph Health Center, East Coast, Demerara	124
Buxton Friendship Health Complex, Buxton, East Coast, Demerara	124
Belview Hospital (Private), Georgetown	108
Prashad Hospital (Private), Thomas and Middle Streets, Georgetown	112
Davis Memorial (Private), Ruimveldt	130
Woodlands Hospital (Private), Carmichael Street, Georgetown	112
Nabaculis Health Center, East Coast, Demerara	136
Plaisance Health Center, Plaisance, East Coast, Demerara	136
Municipal Day Care Center (Creche), South Road, (Side View) Georgetown	138
Lodge Public Health Maternity and Child Care Clinics, Lodge, Hadfield Street, Georgetown	138
Practitioners Medical Centre (Private), Carmichael St., Georgetown	120

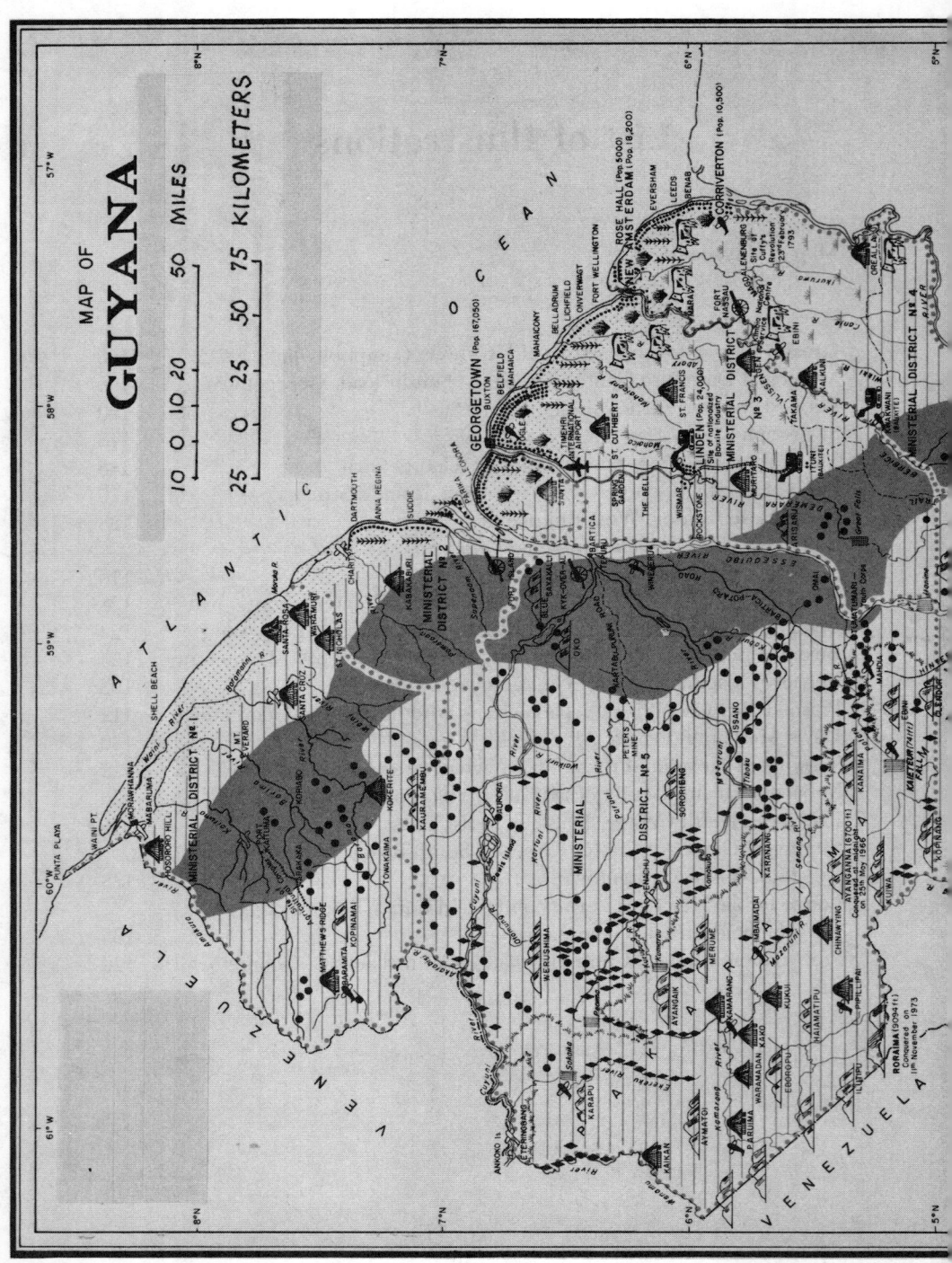

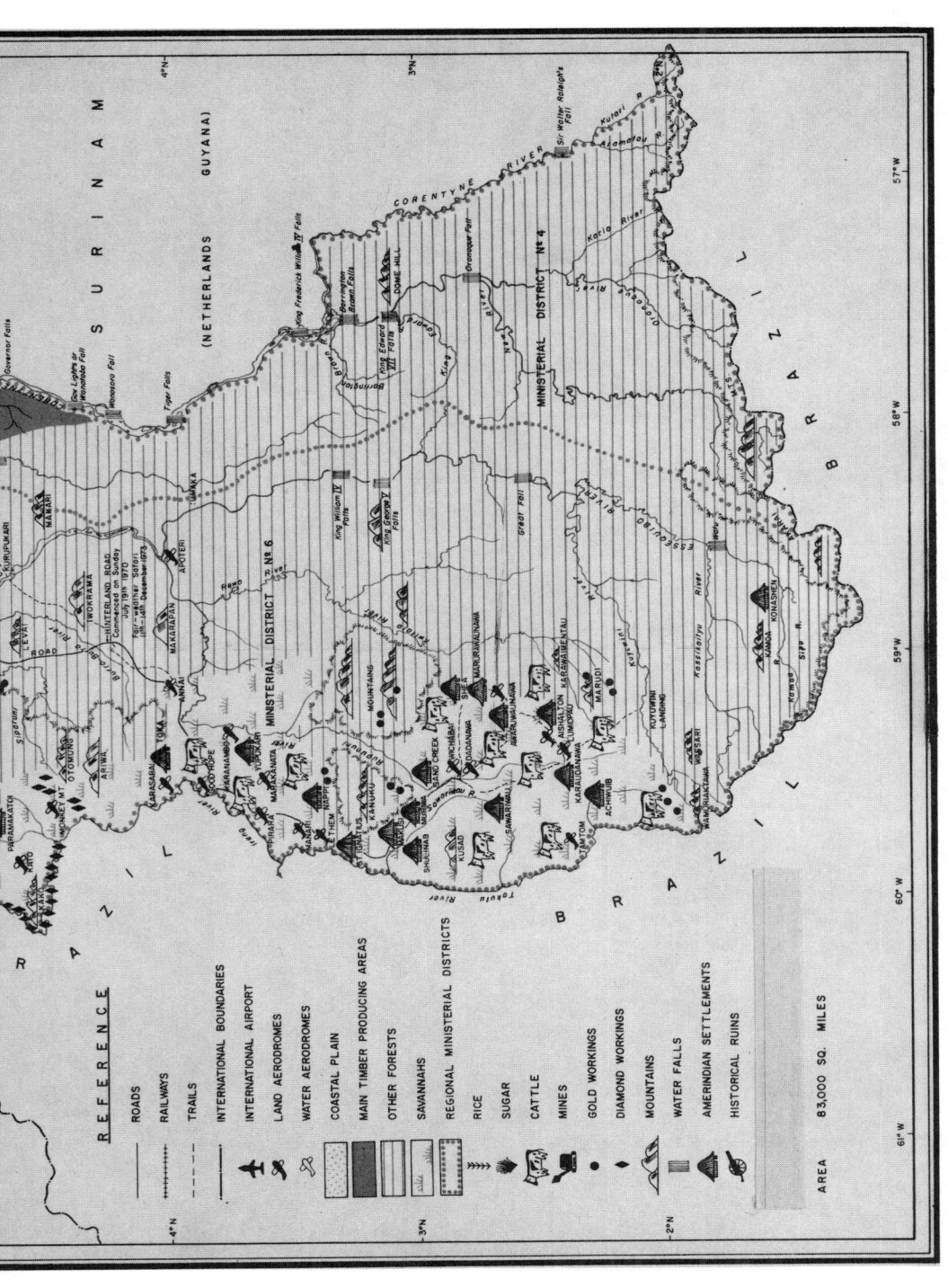

1

Guyana: The Land and Its People

Guyana comprises a total area of 83,000 square miles, being approximately the same size as Great Britain. It is bordered on the north by the Atlantic ocean, on the east by Dutch Guiana (Surinam), on the west by Venezuela, and on the south by Brazil. The history of Guyana has been tortuous. The first Amerindians were believed to have inhabited Guyana as early as 900 A.D., and the area (then called Demerara) was discovered by Europeans during the third voyage of Columbus in 1498.[1] During the sixteenth, seventeenth, and eighteenth centuries, the country changed flags several times as a result of European wars and subsequent treaty negotiations. Guyana has been governed in turn by Spain, Holland, France, and England, each of which made a lasting and significant impact on the culture of Guyana. The most important of these Colonial powers was England, having ruled the then "British Guiana" from 1796 until May 26, 1966, when the country became independent.[2]

The population is composed of several ethnic groups, including Blacks, Portuguese, East Indians, and Chinese. Blacks were brought to Guyana as slaves and now account for approximately 40 percent of the population. The Portugese were invited in from Madeira in 1835, especially for the purpose of increasing the white population of the colony, as many European settlers feared a slave revolt. The first East Indians arrived in Guyana in 1838 as indentured servants,[3] and today they account for 46 per cent of the population. In 1853 there arrived the first Chinese immigrants, who quickly became involved in commerce and small business.[4]

Most of the population lives within a 60-mile-long, 10-mile-deep strip of land along the Atlantic Ocean, between Georgetown, the capital, and New Amsterdam, the second largest city. Bartica and Mackenzie, the bauxite and timber centers, are two small cities of consequence in the interior. It should be remembered that, to most Guyanese, anything south of the highly populated coastal area of the country is usually called "the interior," even though in actual mileage, as related to the size of the country, a given "interior" locale is often relatively close to the ocean.

Guyana means "land of rivers." Huge rivers such as the Essequibo, Marzaruni, Berbice, Corentyne, and Demerara have been important in the historical development of Guyana as well as in the commercial life of the country. Early explorers thought that Guyana was the legendary land of "El Dorado," and they attempted to find cities of gold by exploring the country through its river systems. Guyana is actually rich in gold, diamonds, bauxite, and timber; even today, however, its interior savannahs, jungles, and highlands have yet to be adequately explored or developed. Most of the more populated areas of the country have been given over to sugar, rice, and coconut plantations. Bauxite and sugar are still the leading exports.

The present government is attempting to establish a cooperative socialist country which will be self-sufficient. To this end, many of the businesses that were established under colonialism have been either nationalized or bought by local entrepreneurs. Although Guyana has some of the most beautiful timberland to be found in the world, this resource has not been exploited as an important element of national income. A major difficulty is that many of its woods cannot withstand the hardships of the North American climate. Among the most lucrative local industries are jewelry making, primarily a cottage industry, shirtmaking, and distillation of alcohol. The government has made a concentrated effort to encourage local industry by banning competitive imports and by attempting to develop an appreciation for local products and local cultural values. Nevertheless, many Guyanese have grown accustomed to British and American products, and domestic counterparts seem unappealing. As a result, the black market continues to flourish.

Efforts to improve the cities encounter various kinds of difficulties. Albouystown is known as the "shanty town" area of Georgetown. The socialist Prime Minister, Mr. Forbes Burnham, has met with the inhabitants and spoken about the importance of a clean neighborhood. However, the problem remains, in that, whenever the area has been cleaned up, it soon becomes untidy again. The government's idea is to provide a healthy environment for the children of the community. The mayor of Georgetown along with the city council have taken this campaign seriously.

One of the main problems facing Georgetown is its topographical and geographical location. Because the city is at a low tide level, it has to be protected from the sea. The Georgetown City Council, with the help of the central government, has tackled the problem by instituting a large-scale drainage system which is operated by high-powered electrical pumps. The traditional gravitational drainage system has been converted into a mechanical one which functions rather effectively. To make this system efficient, all the main canals have been deepened by the Hymac machine. However, it is feared that this will create new ecological problems. The dredging creates earthen slopes exposed to erosion, with the result that they may collapse at any time. This problem has already occurred with the canals in Kitty, a village on the east coast of Guyana.

Culture in Guyana

All societies, however large or small, have a culture of their own —the societal way of life, the things that the members of a society think, feel, and do. Culture includes socially transmitted knowledge, beliefs, customs, laws and habits as well as the artifacts of a people.

Culture has a three-fold function: it serves to adapt people to their physical environment through technology, to their group through social organization, and to the supernatural world through religion and magic. General experiences are the same for one particular culture, but differ from culture to culture. As a person grows older, experiences tend to be more numerous and more complex. Thus, every activity exercises a series of influences upon growing numbers of individuals. Although these influences have an effect on cultural personality, they do not create personality.

Society and culture, to some people, seem to be identical; however, they are distinct, though interrelated. Society is an organized group of people, a collection of individuals who live and work together. Culture, on the other hand, is an organized collection of psychic and material factors and of behavioral patterns.

The population of Guyana has not yet reached a million; currently it is about 880,000. Although the British controlled Guyana for almost 150 years, their numbers in Guyana have always been small. Most British who went to Guyana lived within their own group in the colony and returned to England, having only minimal contact with the majority of the people. English culture influenced the Guyanese more directly through the few local people who spent time in England and then returned to the colony.

The Portuguese had a far greater impact on the daily lives of the Guyanese than the English did, because the Portuguese were permanent settlers. There was no plan or thought given to ultimately returning to Madeira or Portugal. Since the Portuguese lived with the other ethnic groups in the colony, they were not isolated in any enclave or ghetto within the Guyanese society. The Roman Catholic Church acted as a basically Portuguese and English institution in the Jesuit tradition, but, as Guyanese became Catholics, they were slowly included within the Portuguese/English/Catholic social milieux.

Most of the members of the black community were Christianized in a variety of formal churches. Thus, throughout the colonial period, one would find it difficult to identify a particular formal institution that would be representative of this large population group. In general, most blacks tended to live in the more urban areas of the country and were represented within all the social groups of Guyana.

East Indians, for the most part, retained their Hindu or Moslem religions and lived on the plantations. The Indian culture became very diluted and weakened. Traditional restrictions concerning food, dress, and interaction between people as practiced in India were relaxed to the point of extinction. Religious ceremonies continued to be performed, although modified to some extent. Much of the original meaning and symbolism of the religions has been forgotten; only some formalized rituals remain.

The extended family systems of India, Africa, and China are still operative in Guyana, but with significant modifications. Family relationships are strong, but families seldom if ever live communally. Individual achievement or disgrace is more of a family matter than it is in other Western countries but is far less important than it is, for example, in India. A similar situation exists in terms of the control and status of older family members in relation to younger family members. What is quite different from India and China is the readiness with which family friends are considered as actual members of the family. It is difficult to judge how permanent the position of the friend is within the family, but, to the casual observer, the relationship would be almost indistinguishable. Children are taught to address their parents' friends as "uncle" and "auntie."

The Chinese population is considerably smaller than that of the black or Indian groups. Most Chinese families run small businesses—groceries, retail shops, and laundries. In recent years, more Chinese have been entering the professions, and the current President of Guyana is Chinese. With the exception of some foods and jewelry designs, traditional Chinese culture has not had a great impact on the overall culture of Guyana.

Food is an important aspect of Guyanese culture. The "good fortune of insuring a return to Guyana" is said to be secured by eating "Labba" (an animal) and drinking creek water. Most Guyanese families have breakfast shortly after sunrise, and work between the end of breakfast and eleven-thirty, when it is time for lunch—the day's main meal. Most women are completely involved with meal preparation. Preparation for tea usually begins at two and continues until around five in the evening. Culturally, the Guyanese diet is as ethnically mixed as is its population. Curry, dahl, rice, and chapati are staples of the diet of all Guyanese. However, chow mein and fried rice are probably eaten at least once a week, as is pepperpot, a beef stew that is the traditional food of the Amerindians.

From Africa, the Guyanese have adopted dishes made with yams, plantain, and cassava such as "metemgee," "fufu" and "dry food." Metemgee is prepared by using coconut milk rather than water in boiling food. This may be rice or such other ground produce as eddoes, yams, or plantains. The British have contributed black cake and black pudding, which is really a sausage, in addition to traditional roasted meat and vegetables. Holiday delicacies such as garlic pork are traditional Portuguese foods.

The traditions surrounding the preparation and eating of food take on enormous cultural proportions and importance in a society where restaurants are few, usually as part of a hotel or private club. In general, people will not eat anything prepared by people they do not know. The food they eat must at least be prepared by people they trust. Food takes on added importance, since one must always be prepared to entertain guests. Keeping in mind that television is banned by the government, people generally visit friends and relatives at least three or four times a week, and parties of all kinds are a way of life.

During special holiday periods such as Christmas and New Year's Day, it is customary for families to visit friends and other relatives more frequently. It is also commonplace for visitors to eat and drink in whatever house they enter. Refusal of food and drink is usually viewed by the host family as being in poor taste. In general, a few words such as "cheers" and "all the best" are expressed by host and guest alike. In such friendly settings, the time is spent in discussing events of the week and the accomplishments of friends and families, and numerous stories are told during which there is laughter and joy.

In formal ceremonies such as weddings, people of all races, ethnic backgrounds, social classes, and creeds come together to celebrate and congratulate the bride and bridegroom. The guests come together in a spirit of oneness, forgetting for a moment that differences and inequalities exist.

In the traditional Hindu weddings, the festivities are usually long, lasting for several days. The bride and bridegroom are usually selected by arrangements made between families. In many instances, the bride's parents will offer a dowry to the bridegroom's parents for the marriage of their daughter. The more educated the bridegroom, the greater the dowry. If the bridegroom is a foreign-educated graduate, the dowry is expected to be greater in amount and quality. The dowry consists of money, gold, diamonds, or perhaps a home for the newlyweds. The arrangements for the dowry are made by a third party who knows the families of the bride and bridegroom. Underlying the dowry system is the idea that the dowry received from the bride's parents is to be used to negotiate a marriage for the sisters of the bridegroom at a future date.

At the completion of the marriage ceremony, the couple returns to the home of the bridegroom's parents. There, the young wife is taught to perform various duties involving the home. Her mother-in-law takes a keen interest in her and, with a watchful eye, supervises the work of her daughter-in-law. Such supervision is intended to teach the new wife to take care of her future home and to "look after" her husband. Within a year, the newlyweds usually find a home of their own.

The socialization process of lower-class children born into Hindu families is unique. The girls are taught rather early to be future homemakers. This training begins in grade school, during which years they are taught to care for younger brothers and sisters while their parents are at work in the rice fields, sugar estates, or gardens of the wealthier families. Formal education for girls in lower-class Hindu families is discouraged by parents since it is the wish of most families that their daughters be married at the earliest possible opportunity. The boys, on the other hand, are told during their grade school years that the only means for social mobility in Guyanese society is success in academic work. A son is protected from doing other activities so that his time can be spent studying Guyanese history, poetry, mathematics, and foreign languages. It is very common for Hindu families to invest all of their life savings in the education of a son as a possible physician or lawyer.

Children of the middle and upper classes are encouraged to educate themselves to the maximum. Parents assist by arranging tutors to teach their children after the regular school session. Girls are encouraged to learn music at a very early age, while boys in grade school learn extracurricular activities such as cricket and soccer. It is the hope of parents in these classes that their daughters will "marry well" and that their sons will become future physicians or lawyers. These are common aspirations of parents for their children in Guyanese society.

In an attempt to create an egalitarian society, the government has nationalized all training institutions so completely that boys and girls of all social classes now must attend and be taught in the same classrooms. Education is compulsory, so it is less likely that girls will be denied equal opportunities and privileges to be educated as they have been in the past.

From a cultural point of view, hospitality plays a very important role in the society. Relatives, friends, and foreign visitors are greeted warmly and are always welcome to share meals with the host family. Arrangements are usually made to accommodate families and friends for several days without thought of monetary return. If the host families cannot provide the necessary accommodations, then other families and friends are consulted and in all instances guests have a home in which to enjoy themselves and to stay as long as they wish. The longer the guests remain in the home, the greater is the satisfaction of the host family.

In a culture such as that of Guyana, illness is viewed with fear. If an individual must undergo surgery, the condition is viewed seriously, as surgery is considered the final decision to save the patient from death. If the patient survives the surgery, the patient is told that a "strong heart" is responsible for the success of the operation. In the recovery stage, families and friends will visit regularly and they will bring various foods, fruits, and delicacies without the knowledge of the nurses or attending physician. Very few inquiries are made by friends as to whether or not a restricted diet has been scheduled for the patient.

During visits by friends and relatives, the patient will be kept informed of the latest news in the villages, towns, and estates along the east and west margins of the country. Visitors will announce the most recent scores in cricket matches and will narrate vivid descriptions to the sick person. The purpose of communicating with the sick person in such a fashion is to "take the mind off the illness."

It is also of interest to note that, in a culture such as that of Guyana, it is customary for relatives and friends visiting a patient in a hospital to talk with other sick persons and visit with them, even though the parties have never met previously. Sick individuals and acquaintances in a hospital ward quickly establish a marvelous rapport among themselves, as if they had known each other for several years. A conversation will result, and inquiries will be made about the patient's illness, how the illness occurred, the attending physician's name, the quality of the food, whether or not families and friends have visited, and the tentative dismissal date of the patient from the hospital. Thus, irrespective of race, social class, or creed, the Guyanese people are very sympathetic to the ill person. Feelings of empathy are generated by the visitor toward the sick individual. The patient is encouraged to get well and to return to the daily routine of work and recreation as quickly as possible. Thus, sickness in the hospital setting in Guyanese culture is viewed as a communal affair in which society wants the patient out of the sick role as soon as possible.

The Political Situation

The political institution of a society is a social and cultural system establishing formal methods for obtaining and exercising power within a given domain through agencies which have legitimate authority.

Power is the ability or potential ability to influence the behavior and/or thoughts of others. Power can be analyzed on two levels, namely, authority and influence.

Authority is legitimate power which stems from an office or position of status in the social structure of society. Influence is power that is based upon personality attributes of the person who has the power and of those whom he influences.

Political parties in Guyana have developed, and continue to develop, with definite and diverse platforms. The main parties are: "The Peoples' Progressive Party" (PPP), "The Peoples' National Congress" (PNC), and "The United Front" (UF).

The period from 1891 to 1928 was one of economic change, with the sugar industry going through a series of depressions. In 1917, when the indentured labor supply from India stopped, that source of cheap labor was abruptly and totally cut off. Those Indians who stayed in Guyana, but were no longer under indenture, turned to cultivating rice independently rather than sugar on plantations. Britain became dissatisfied because the colony was losing money.

In 1928, the British gave Guyana a new constitution. The Courts of Policy and the Combined Courts, which were the former policy bodies, were replaced by the Legislative Council consisting of 15 members appointed by the government (all Europeans) and 14 members elected by the people (Africans and Asians). The Guyanese, however, continued to show their opposition to British domination. Agitation led to yet another new constitution in 1945, which provided for a Legislative Council with a Governor, a Colonial Secretary, a Financial Secretary, an Attorney General, and five elected members. The franchise was given to all literate persons over 21 years of age who were tenants of three acres of land or who owned land valued at $120. In 1946, Dr. Cheddi Jagan, American-educated dentist, along with his American wife Janet, formed the Political Committee and was elected to the Legislative Council. In 1948, Mr. Forbes Burnham, British-educated barrister-at-law, the present Prime Minister of Guyana, joined Dr. Jagan's political movement; both were dissatisfied with British control of Guyana. Their joint efforts resulted in the creation of the People's Progressive Party, in 1949, which sought self-government based on economic development and social revolution.

In 1953, Guyana again received a new constitution. This constitution, based on universal suffrage, provided for a Legislative and Executive Council comprised of the Governor, three ex-officio members, 24 elected members from the State Council, and six members from the House of Assembly. On April 27, 1953, the PPP, led by Dr. Jagan and Mr. Burnham, won 18 of 24 seats. There ensued various strikes on sugar plantations during September 1953. In response, the PPP prepared to pass legislation in support of the strikers—they supported a Guyana Industrial Workers Union. The British government responded by suspending the constitution and calling in troops from Jamaica. On October 20, 1953, a White Paper was released condemning the subversive methods used by Dr. Jagan. On

February 18, 1954, Dr. Jagan was arrested and imprisoned for six months. Shortly afterwards, in 1955, the PPP split; Dr. Jagan and Burnham found agreement impossible. There was relative calm in Guyana between 1955 and 1960; the PPP was in power and maintained ties with the Colonial Office in England. A constitutional conference on British Guiana was held in London in March 1960, and it was decided that Guyana would become independent sometime in the future. In 1961, the country was given internal self-government, but this was not enough because "real power to govern, to carry out our program fully was withheld from us throughout. We were in office but not in power . . . constitutionally. We were simply advisors to him [the British governor]."[5]

In 1961, Dr. Jagan's cabinet (he had been elected with 42.6 percent of the vote) announced new taxes. The people began to protest the new taxes, and the government responded by prohibiting public assembly. It was not until after violent riots in 1962 that Dr. Jagan withdrew his tax scheme. Another Constitutional Conference on British Guiana was held in London, October 26–November 6, 1962, resulting in a proposal of proportional membership in 1966 with the voting age remaining 21. The country at that time was under the leadership of Mr. Forbes Burnham, head of the PNC and the present Prime Minister. Dr. Jagan's voice was never silent; he greeted "the idea of such independence" with harshness. He realized that national liberation did not necessarily imply political independence alone. There was an inherent danger of becoming nothing more than a colony of the mother country.[6]

Dr. Jagan advocated total independence from Britain and "other" states, interpreted as a reference to the United States. In 1966, Guyana's economic life was dominated by Britain and North America. Britain owned 100 per cent of the sugar industry, while Canada and the United States controlled the mining of bauxite. The U.S. also controlled the mining of manganese. In addition, banking, insurance, shipping, and foreign and local wholesale trade were virtually all under foreign control.

Although Guyana became independent on May 26, 1966, it continued to maintain strong ties with the "mother country." In 1966, nevertheless, Dr. Jagan condemned the surviving Western imperialism. In 1969, the government, headed by Mr. Burnham (he had been elected in 1964), made a move which would "sever" Guyana's ties with this imperialism.

The change into a Republic was relatively simple. The Governor General, the head of state, was replaced by a President of Guyana, a citizen, qualified for membership in the National Assembly. However, in terms of power, his position was similar to that of the governor. Guyana became a Cooperative Republic in 1970. Guyana, however, was not an ordinary republic. Its ideology was based to a great degree on socialism. It was perhaps in this spirit of "cooperation" that the government wished to lessen the racial tensions and conflicts which had long been a part of Guyanese society. The two major political parties corresponded with the largest ethnic and racial groups, the PPP being predominantly East Indian and the PNC, predominantly African. Voting was based on the idea of "apanjaht," the Hindu word for "vote for you own kind."

In a later address at a May Day rally, Dr. Cheddi Jagan pledged his "critical" support for the PNC platform. He said that he wanted unity and struggle to be their guide: unity in defense of their territorial integrity, and struggle against the enemy within and outside the country. Mr. Burnham welcomed the pledge of cooperation by Dr. Jagan and hoped that, even though there were differences between them, they had many more areas of agreement. He also knew that any division would weaken their mutually held position of opposition to colonial status for Guyana.

Summary

Guyana was a former colony of Spain, Holland, France, and England. It became independent on May 26, 1966. The Guyanese population is a heterogeneous one. There are blacks from Africa, East Indians from India, Chinese, and European-descent whites. Like all colonial countries, Guyana has imitated life styles, languages, and other aspects of various material cultures.

The Portuguese had a far greater impact on the life of the Guyanese than did the English because the Portuguese were permanent settlers. Most of the black members in the community were Christianized, while East Indians, for the most part, retained their Hindu or Moslem religion as well as their basic cultural heritage. The Chinese culture had virtually no impact on the overall culture of Guyana.

Guyana has a long political history. Britain helped the people to shape the Guyanese constitution. The British gave Guyana a new constitution in 1928, 1945, and again in 1953. In March 1960, a constitutional conference on British Guiana was held in London and it was decided that Guyana should be given freedom. Today, there are three political parties: the Peoples' Progressive Party (PPP); the Peoples' National Congress (PNC); and the United Front (UF). Presently, the government is headed by Mr. Forbes Burnham, who is trying to move the government closer to socialism through cooperatives. The socio-economic and political situation will help us to understand some background factors of the health care system in Guyana.

2

Health Services

History of the Georgetown Hospital

During the eighteenth century, the population of Guyana was predominantly black. The few Europeans were overseers on plantations, attached to military units posted there, or employed in government service. The first hospitals were part of military posts and were administered by a surgeon major. One such early military hospital was in the Stabroek Ward on the site now occupied by the museum. The ward received its name because Stabroek was the thriving sugar plantation that emerged later as the capital city of Georgetown. This military hospital served only people in the government and military services. The remaining persons were sent to a "yaws house" (named after an infectious disease of the tropics) which occupied a site at the rear of the Stabroek Ward located in Brickdam, near the present Ministry of Health buildings.

In the nineteenth century, the Stabroek military hospital became a colonial hospital, while yaws houses continued to serve leprosy and infectious cases. In the twentieth century yaws houses were thatched houses, in ruinous condition, described by Dr. J. W. Dunkin as "miserable hovels." These yaws houses were also known as "pest houses." Even the colonial hospital was far from satisfactory, and in 1808, Surgeon Major Tuies addressed a letter to the authorities stating that he had repeatedly sent letters to petition for the "alleviation of the sufferings of the wretched beings under his care without any results." The authorities were indignant at what they termed "highly improper and disrespectful language." For these allegedly unfounded and disparaging reflections on the hospital, he was dismissed at once and Dr. J. W. Dunkin was appointed in his place.

Shortly after, repeated complaints were made by various persons concerning disturbances within the hospital. Thomas Frankland finally submitted a complaint, in 1918, regarding the nuisance caused by noise from psychiatric patients. This complaint received attention, and, in the same year, a red brick building for psychiatric patients was erected near the hospital. This building was used for many years and various purposes before a fire destroyed it in 1945.

An outbreak of yellow fever occurred in the colony in 1837, and a serious problem arose in recruiting sailors to work on vessels enroute to

British Guiana because of the lack of hospital accommodations in the colony for sick seamen. In August of that year, a house was rented near Urquharg's Stelling to be used to care for sick sailors, but this temporary building never proved to be satisfactory. By 1838, the people in charge of the hospitals were discontented over the conditions of the medical facilities, and they determined to make improvements. The Combined Court voted to appoint a committee to erect a colonial and seamen's hospital. Following the Committee's report, an ordinance was passed to provide medical aid for seamen. In 1844, 300 beds were provided for the colonial hospital. A general hospital with an outpatient department was also started. The year 1844 marked the beginning of immigration into Guyana, one year after the emancipation of slaves throughout the colonial empire. Four years later, in 1848, a building (formerly a coffee shop) and a portion of the surrounding land were acquired for a seamen's hospital.

The seamen's colonial and psychiatric hospitals were merged in 1850, marking the start of the present Public Hospital. About 25 years ago, the present seamen's ward replaced the original seamen's hospital, now Georgetown Hospital, and only one original building still remains. This is the L-shaped building now standing at the corner of Thomas and Middle Streets within the hospital compound.[1]

Health Care Developments: 1933–1966

Dr. George Giglioli, retired medical advisor to the Sugar Producers' Association and honorary government malariaologist, laid the basic foundations for the eradication of malaria by means of a very skillfully designed scheme of house-spraying with DDT.

On June 28, 1966, Dr. Giglioli gave a striking and remarkable analysis of health care on the sugar estates prior to the independence of Guyana. His views were given on Radio Demerara. Dr. Giglioli noted:

> I had been in Guyana for ten years when, in November 1933, I started working on the sugar estates. After Mackenzie, it was like moving into an entirely new country.
>
> At Mackenzie, nothing was old, and the Plant seemed to get newer every day; on the estates, most things appeared old and dingy, shabby, and in disrepair. The ranges, in which most of the population lived, and hospitals were particularly dilapidated and unsightly; the equipment, ranges of drugs, and standards of treatment offered within the hospital were consonant with their general appearance.
>
> To understand this deplorable situation, a brief digression may be necessary.

The ranges and the hospitals were built mostly in the past century, on standard specifications laid down by the Colonial Government in consultation with the Government of India; they were intended for the housing of immigrants who came to this country on 5-year contracts. These buildings are subject to periodical inspection by the Government. The estates were bound to make work available for the immigrants and also free housing in the ranges, and provide free medical assistance; they supplied the hospital, the drugs, the dispensers, and the nurses. The hospitals, however, came under the jurisdiction of the District Government Medical Officer who visits them three times a week and attends to patients free of charge.

Indentured immigration came to an end in 1917, and, by 1922, all outstanding contracts were reciprocal; legal obligations between immigrants and planters thus ceased to exist. The immigrants who did not return to India were free to move out and seek work elsewhere; the planters, on the other hand, had no obligation to provide housing and medical treatment, and were not required to keep their ranges and hospital in good repair.

In Trinidad, the immigrants rapidly moved off the estates, and into the villages; the ranges and hospitals also disappeared at an early date. On the Guyana coastlands, however, agricultural land had to be protected by sea defenses, drained, and irrigated; outside the estates and the established villages, there was little or no land available. Immigrants and planters thus took the line of least resistance: the immigrants remained on the estates where work was available, and they continued to occupy the ranges free of charge with the consent of the planters, who also continued to give free medical treatment, while the District-General Medical Officer went on visiting the hospitals three times a week as in the past. Thus nothing changed, except that arrangements were on a basis of mutual interest and had no legal foundation; moreover, the obligation to maintain the ranges and hospitals had lapsed, and, during the depression of the 1920's, little or no money was available for this purpose. Thus, deterioration set in at a very rapid pace, and, with every year that passed, the problem of re-housing the estate population became more urgent and its solution more difficult.

The water situation was as shocking as that of housing: drinking water was drawn from the so-called "sweet-water canals," which got their supply from the general irrigation network and were often situated at only a few yards from the sidelines, over which the communal latrines were built. During droughts, the water became low and stagnant, and during the rains, with extensive flooding of the range yards, they became massively contaminated.

In the late twenties and early thirties, the low prices of sugar and the shortage of labor caused a number of estates to go out of cultivation;

first, Hampton Court, then Anna Regina and Marianville in Essequibo and Providence were similarly menaced.

In November 1933, I joined Davison's Sugar Estate—Blairmont, Providence and Bath. It was hoped that, by improving health conditions, the flow of young people off the estates might be stopped, and that others from the outside might be attracted to seek residence, and therefore work, on these plantations.

Health conditions at Blairmont in 1933 were appalling; there were only 1900 residents at the time, but, in the first month after my arrival, there were no less than 11 deaths, 5 from extreme anemia in young expectant mothers. Malaria was rampant and grave, as malaria mosquito production, and therefore malaria transmission, continued at all seasons.

On this background of malaria saturation, the effects of malnutrition were magnified, particularly in expectant mothers, often giving rise to grave and fatal anemia. Torpid ulcers of the legs were extremely prevalent and disabling; they too were due to the combined effects of chronic malaria, malnutrition, and neglect. Pneumonia, bronchitis, and other chronic lung conditions caused much suffering, and were often fatal.

We began by rebuilding the hospital, adding a wing for children and a clinical laboratory; the range of drugs was extended and treatment modernized. The hospital diet was changed to cope with the prevalence of malnutrition, and methods were introduced to ensure that outpatients should take their treatment as prescribed.

In spite of the fact that in the early 1930's all of the wonder drugs of today were not even dreamed of, we reaped immediate and remarkable results; by the end of 1936, the third year of our experiment, the population of Blairmont had increased by 7.7 per cent; death had fallen by 24 per cent, and births had increased by 11 per cent; hospitalization for malaria had fallen greatly, and grave anemia of pregnancy and chronic leg ulcers had all but disappeared; the infant mortality per 1000 live births had fallen from 206 in 1934 to 85.7 in 1936. Finally, the average weight of infants at birth had increased by over one pound. Particularly important were advances made at Blairmont in the study of malaria epidemiology and transmission, between 1933 and 1937—with these we shall, however, deal at a later stage.

These Blairmont results proved so encouraging that, in 1937, Bookers asked me to establish a Central Medical Control Laboratory for the purpose of imposing health conditions on all sugar estates. Here it soon became evident that the public health measures then available applied to the estates only and not to the neighboring villages, and, though they were costly, would yield only negligible results.

A reorganization of methods of treatment would, on the contrary, produce immediate benefit as had been demonstrated practically at Blairmont. This, however, involved a complete recasting of medical services. There were, at the time, 21 estate hospitals in the country, all of them of deplorable standard. This large number had been justified at the time of mule-and-buggy transportation; it was ridiculous and unnecessarily expensive in the age of the motor ambulance. A single hospital in each district would be adequate, and, if it were properly designed, equipped, and staffed and motor ambulances were made available, much better services could be rendered. Early in 1938, I submitted proposals for a reorganization of medical services on the sugar estates. This project was favorably received, but, pending the then imminent visit by the West India Royal Commission, it was decided to postpone any definite decision until the findings and recommendations of the Commission became available.

War broke out in 1939, and the Commission's report was not released until 1944; by that time, many other difficulties caused my project to be shelved.

Meanwhile, however, the investigations on the epidemiology of malaria, which had been so fruitful at Blairmont, were intensified and extended; in 1939, a Malaria Research Unit was established jointly by the government, the sugar industry, and the Rockefeller Foundation. Mr. Ramjattan followed me as a Chief Field Technician. My work at this state was interrupted by war, as I was interned at H.M.P.S. for 26 months. Here too, however, I was able to continue investigations on some aspects of malaria epidemiology, and these studies paid dividends, some years later, in shaping policies for the maintenance of malaria eradication on the coastlands.

After my return to the Sugar Estates in 1945, while directing the DDT anti-malaria campaign, a detailed survey of the estate housing situation was made, so that this information was available when the Venn Commission carried out its investigation of the sugar industry in 1948. The Commission found that the sugar estates should be responsible for the re-housing of the bulk of the estate population still living in the even more dilapidated ranges. Government, however, ruled that re-housing of estate workers should be financed through the Sugar Industry Labor Welfare Fund. This has been done. The numerous, well-laid out new housing areas aggregate over 10,000 houses, which have blossomed throughout the sugar belt, with their large lots, neat houses, piped potable water supply, paved roads, playing fields, and recreation halls. They are the eloquent proof of this great effort, carried out entirely with funds earned from the production of sugar.

The Venn Commission also examined recommendations for the reorganization and centralization of hospital assistance. While agreeing with this concept, they found that hospitalization was a function of government, and they recommended that a number of rural state hospitals should be erected for the care of both villagers and estate residents, also for the purpose of alleviating the heavy burden carried by the Georgetown hospital. Government, however, after some delay on this very important matter, finally decided to build health centers only, but not rural hospitals. In the meanwhile, on the estates, we proceeded to implement the Venn Commission's recommendations as far as was in our power; most of the obsolete, dilapidated hospitals were demolished. Only five remained along with one regional estate hospital. These conditions existed pending the erection of several state hospitals by the government.

This reorganization was greatly facilitated by the eradication of malaria from the coastlands between 1945 and 1951, as estate morbidity had been drastically reduced and most of the hospitals stood empty. This, however, was only temporary; the extension of Workmen's Compensation to agricultural workers in 1947, altered the nature of medical practice on the sugar estates. The District-General Medical Officers who were still responsible for the medical care of estate laborers on the basis of regulations introduced during the last century, found themselves swamped by patients claiming compensation; most of these claims were genuine, many were serious. The General Medical Officers argued, rightly so, that this new work could not be regarded as pertaining to their established duties; some refused to see such cases, and the estate medical services became badly disrupted. This proved the final factor in bringing about the adoption of my 1948 proposal for an independent Sugar Estate Medical Service; such a service came into operation at the end of 1952.

Today, the industry employs six full-time Medical Officers; it has a well-equipped central hospital at Lusignan provided with first-class x-ray apparatus and a clinical laboratory. In addition, there are twenty-one new dispensaries on the estate, and of these, seventeen have emergency wards. A fleet of eight ambulances provides for the rapid transportation of patients.

The Sugar Estate Medical Service effectively provides for the medical care of 84,300 estate workers and their dependents; that is equivalent to a little more than one-fifth of Guyana's coastal rural population.

The sugar industry has come a very long way during the past thirty-three years, and living conditions on the estates have been dramatically revolutionized. In my mind, the rapid conversion of this ancient and traditionally bound industry to modern scientific methods and advances is everywhere evident—in the fields, in the factories, in the hospitals, and in the dispensaries.[2]

Structure of Present-day Health Services

The government of Guyana, in a 1966-1977 Statement of Development Program, was determined to secure for the nation the highest possible level of social welfare.[3] Accordingly, the expansion and improvement of the health services were approved social objectives, viewed as prerequisites for economic development. Thus, the entire structure of the health services and their expansion was planned as an integral part of the Development Program.

At the government level, health facilities are divided into two broad groups: curative and preventive. The dispensaries, public hospitals, and district cottage hospitals practice curative medicine. Preventive medicine includes all aspects of work done on environmental sanitation, i.e., inspection of food, maternal and child welfare. The chief administration offices of the Health Ministry are the Central Board of Health (Statutory), of which the Chief Medical Officer is Chairman, and the Ministry of Health, administered by the Chief Medical Officer who is the Technical and Administrative Advisor.

Preventive Medicine

The following subsections discuss the state of medical development in treatment of the most common serious diseases in Guyana.

Malaria

At the moment, the country has eradicated malaria on the coastal plain and strong efforts are continually being made to do the same in the hinterland. This success is the result of international agencies working with local personnel in Guyana. A three-pronged method was developed consisting of examination of blood slides, treatment with chloroquinized salt, and spraying DDT. Most malaria cases are reported from the interior. The eradication of malaria has saved lives and eliminated lost days of work for the people of this country. It is true that an initial increase in the crude birth rate, along with a decline in the crude death rate, had been to a large extent due to the elimination of malaria.

Filaria

Filaria is still a serious medical problem in Guyana, and thousands of hours are lost every year among the workers. A side effect is the disruption of homes and care of children when mothers are afflicted with this debilitating disease. Filariasis, as a worm infestation disease of the blood and tissues, affects the legs and breasts in females and the legs and scrotum in males. A pilot program, in operation since September 1955, has proven itself inadequate to solve this problem in the country.

Pulmonary Tuberculosis

Developments in both curative and preventive medicine against pulmonary tuberculosis have been very successful as evidenced by the number of now empty beds in the tuberculosis sanatorium. All campaigns in the rural areas and hinterlands are presently being stepped up. The disease is still active among the Amerindians. Since it is difficult to provide ambulatory treatment for those afflicted in their remote homelands, they are kept in hospitals until cured of the disease.

Maternal and Child Welfare Clinics

For the years 1954 and 1955, the principal cause of death were diseases in early infancy. Maternal and child death rates for these years were 149.7 and 146.0 per 100,000 population, respectively. The following vital services are provided at 33 health centers and 112 maternal and child health clinics dispersed over the rural areas: a) nutrition (milk and milk products, vitamin supplements); b) immunization (diphtheria, whooping cough, antipoliomyelitis and small pox); c) social disease programs at pre-natal clinics, including treatment for mothers showing positive contact, tracing and treatment of husbands; and d) curative and preventive treatment of pre-school children. These services have contributed, in large measure, to the decline in the infant mortality rate. Continuous improvement of services will reinforce this favorable trend.

Environmental Sanitation Program

The Environmental Sanitation Program was introduced in 1960 and emphasized the importance of a potable water supply and adequate feces disposal in order to stop the breeding of insect vectors and bacteria, to reduce typhoid, filaria, gastroenteritis, and dysentery, as well as to stop the spread of parasitic diseases such as hookworm and other worm infestations. The project started in Essequibo, where the parasitic infestation of children and adults was about 80 per cent to 90 per cent, with hookworm alone having a rate of 65 per cent. This program will reduce the anemia which goes along with hookworm.

Typhoid

Typhoid fever, or enteric fever, is endemic in Guyana, and epidemics are common in the rural areas. Contamination occurs through water and food, and, in every epidemic, the "culprit" is always a carrier. The figures for 1963 and 1964 could be considered low if compared with previous years (see Table 4, p. 149). According to the Medical Research Council, it is undetermined whether the favorable trend was the result of improved sanitation. It may also have been the result of immunity given to school-age children through typhoid vaccine trials.

Curative Medicine

Curative medicine is practiced in the hospitals and district centers. Hospitals have differing amounts of equipment and staffing and the cottage hospitals are often inadequately staffed, lacking equipment for diagnosis or research. The Georgetown Hospital is the only one in Guyana which can really be called a "hospital" by international standards; the others do not measure up to this district's performance in comparison with overseas territories. The improvement of these other hospitals will provide better treatment for the public. Presently, people are leaving areas where the poorly equipped hospitals are located to travel to the public hospital in Georgetown for treatment, thereby increasing the load of an already overcrowded facility.

Proposals

The government has indicated that the proposals listed in this development plan are intended to assist in the smoother running of the health services by providing better hospital facilities, i.e., research investigations and treatment as well as better coordination of district and central services.

Building on the existing structure will cause greater health benefits to the nation. Since there was no true planning involved in the growth of the present structure of health services, original planning and extensive reorganization of the entire structure are greatly needed but often very difficult. Now that the Marshall Plan for local government reform is being considered for implementation, it should be helpful to identify the rural medicine districts subdivided into areas:

Medical District	Number of Areas
Essequibo	3
Essequibo Islands	2
East Demerara	4
West Demerara	3
East Berbice	5
West Berbice	1

The government has indicated that the health services should be reorganized as a three-tier pyramid. At the first level, there will be varying numbers of health centers in each area, with the exception of the Essequibo Islands district. All dispensaries, health clinic centers, and cottage hospitals (to be renamed "health centers") will be directly supervised by the Chief Medical Officer. They will serve as multi-purpose units providing facilities for maternal and child welfare work, including environmental sanitation, health education, public health nursing, control of communicable disease, treatment of minor medical and surgical conditions, family planning, and midwifery. These facilities will be responsible for all health activities in the areas they serve.

It is clear that few of the present centers are capable of providing for all of the departments listed above. They are to be reviewed with the objective of providing the following minimum accommodations: a) consulting/examination room; b) treatment/dressing room with facilities for minor surgery; c) storage room for records, welfare goods, drugs and dressings, public health and health education equipment, and supplies, and d) where local conditions make it necessary, "wards" for eight to ten patients whose conditions do not warrant transfer to a hospital but who should be kept under observation for a few days. Also, there will be midwifery facilities, each consisting of a delivery room and two to six lying-in beds and kitchen facilities.

The responsibility of administrative district local authorities will be the upkeep of all health centers. In reorganization, it is imperative that such centers be properly located in consideration of such factors as population density, lines of communication, etc. Careful review of the existing centers, which constitute the other two tiers of health care services, is therefore necessary.

District Hospitals

The second highest level of health delivery services is made up of the district hospitals. There should be at least one well-equipped hospital within the designated area of each district to provide facilities for diagnosis and treatment of all medical, surgical, gynecological, obstetrical, and infectious diseases. In order to afford every medical officer the opportunity to practice medicine with modern facilities, every hospital will be equipped with the following: a) an operating theater; b) adequate general facilities; c) pre-natal, post-natal, and child health clinics; d) x-ray facilities; e) laboratory facilities capable of all routine microscopic and biochemical investigations; and f) adequate mortuary and autopsy facilities.

There must, of necessity, be adequate facilities for transportation at the disposal of both health centers and district hospitals. The remarks made on siting, in connection with health centers, should apply also to district hospitals, although there are only a few which may seem to fit in automatically, e.g., Suddie Hospital for the Essequibo Coast and Islands, Mabaruma Hospital for the North West District, etc.

The seven-year development plan provides for a number of improvements and extensive alterations to individual hospitals as well as for varying services to other hospitals. It is important to realize that, before these works can begin to be useful, they must be considered in the light of the proposed reorganization of the health services. Some recommendations are: a) renovation and improvement of Mabaruma Hospital by providing an adequate operating theater and x-ray facilities, improved outpatient facilities, improved kitchen, laundry, and storage areas as well as provision of new ward space for approximately 12 tuberculosis patients; b) improvement of New Amsterdam Hospital by providing for a new outpatient department, a new maternal and child welfare clinic, and a new laundry area with an elevator; c) improvement in psychiatric services by providing an intensive care unit with a central admission and treatment center; d) completion of extensions to Lethem Hospital in the Rupununi; e) building a new theatre block at the Georgetown Hospital; f) planning and completing of phase I of a General Reference Program; and g) improvement of extensions to other medical units.

New Georgetown Hospital

On the third level will be the general reference hospital, which is to be staffed by specialists with ample supporting medical and auxiliary staff. Cases requiring specialized care will be separated from those which can be treated adequately in district hospitals by a competent practitioner. It is here that the medical staff will be trained at the intern level, and even at a higher level, with the long-range goal of their working in district hospitals as potential specialists. This hospital will contain the following departments: a) self-contained obstetric department, particularly designed to deal with abnormal deliveries, b) x-ray department of three radio diagnostic rooms, c) operating suite comprising operating theatres with central sterilizing facilities, endoscopy room, a room for removing plasters, and another for procedures involving overt septic cases, d) comprehensive consultant out-patient department with specialized services, e.g., opthalmology, ear-nose-throat, etc., e) full laboratory service including mortuary and post-mortem facilities, which will provide pathology services for the hospital and also carry out all the more involved and difficult investigations for the whole country, f) physiotherapy unit, g) kitchen and staff dining rooms, h) residential accommodation for junior medical staff, i) training school for nurses and ancillary staff, j) residential accommodation for nursing staff, k) medical library, specialists' sitting room, seminar rooms, and l) hospital administrative offices.

This is the development which the health services of Guyana will be striving to achieve for a number of years. It will be most beneficial if communicable disease can be treated more effectively at the local level. Special services for such conditions as mental illness, leprosy, and tuberculosis will also be improved.

Leprosy (Hansen's Disease)

Leprosy will continue to be treated at the Mahaica Hospital. A detailed analysis will be given later.

Tuberculosis

Adequate treatment for tuberculosis will take place at district hospitals. The only patients to be transferred to the general reference hospitals will be those with special problems. Patients will be transported to their district hospital periodically for assessment and x-rays through the provision of better and more adequate facilities in the hinterlands. Amerindians will be hospitalized in their own areas rather than being transferred to Best Hospital for extended periods of time.

It may be possible that mentally ill patients who are released after brief treatment can be cared for in the vicinity of Georgetown—at Best Hospital—while those requiring a longer period of treatment will be provided for in the intensive care unit of the general hospital. Long-term patients and others with virtually no possibility of ever being discharged will most likely be housed at the existing psychiatric hospital which will be renovated.

Services for the Hinterland

The hinterland includes the North West—8,500 square miles, Upper Mazaruni and Guyuni—21,525 square miles, and Rupununi—40,000 square miles. There is one doctor stationed at Mabaruma, North West District, none in the Mazaruni, and one at Lethem, Rupununi. Servicing the whole of the Upper Mazaruni District are several dispensaries and one nursing station at Kamarang. There is a need for some detailed planning for each of these areas to insure development of both preventive and curative health services such as a reduction of infant mortality and morbidity, maternity and child health facilities, and a proper system of excreta disposal and distribution of pure water.

A high incidence of the following diseases still exists: tuberculosis, gastroenteritis, anemia, yaws, hookworm, and other worm infections. Also, there is an urgent need for higher quality dental services in all areas. It will not be possible to follow closely the reorganizational pattern for the coastlands due to the major problem of transportation. However, it may be possible to build some comprehensive health centers in many village centers.

Geriatric Unit

Since many elderly patients have long term illnesses that are never totally cured but only somewhat alleviated, a geriatric unit will be built. Gerontology has become an important part of Western European medicine. Placed in this unit will be all of the inoperable cancer patients. Specialists in geriatrics will serve to make life less burdensome to patients with these illnesses. The number of beds for the unit will depend on the bed space at the district hospital.

Community Aid in Health Services Development

In light of all the hospital facilities to be erected or altered, it is important to involve the community in all aspects of the work. Cost of these projects can be reduced if volunteer groups of young men and women provide their labor. These savings from volunteer labor then will be reallocated to other departments where funds are needed for development. It is thought that in every district the community will realize its responsibilities and assist in the formation of its health services.

The General Development Plan for Guyana's Health Services

The general plan includes an examination and reorganization of the existing health centers, child and maternity welfare centers, and all cottage hospitals and dispensaries in accord with the needs of the individual areas. Also included in the plan are new and improved equipment and health facilities for district hospitals. The Georgetown Hospital will undergo reorganization so as to function as a district hospital. Also, in Georgetown, a general reference hospital is to be built.

The new work will occur in five stages. Stage one will consist of alterations at Best Hospital, upgrading of Lethem Hospital, rehabilitation and expansion of Mabaruma Hospital, and building of a new theatre block at Georgetown Hospital. Stage two involves improvements of Skelton, New Amsterdam, and Suddie Hospitals. Stage three involves the reorganization of Georgetown Hospital. Stage four involves rehabilitation of Fort Canje Hospital, and stage five encompasses completion of all plans and drawings for the proposed general reference hospital.

Anticipated Results

Fourteen million dollars is the anticipated expenditure for this seven-year development plan. For such complete change and renovation of a nation's health plan, this is not a large sum. Unless it is very well planned, the development will not improve services. In the long run, it is projected that existing facilities are to be used to the full extent.

Dr. B. E. C. Hopwood, Health and Manpower consultant from the Commonwealth Secretariat, has discussed with the Caribbean territory health authorities his plans to arrange for a grant from the Agency for International Development (AID). Such a grant will be used for training health personnel. Dr. Hopwood requested the regional health offices to concentrate on research in diabetes and hypertension.

A group of doctors and professionals is trying to establish "The International College of Naturopathy and Applied Sciences" in Guyana. If it materializes, it will be the first of its kind in South America and the Caribbean. The Institute will experiment with herbs to produce medicine and drugs in hope of curing syphilis, cancer and other diseases. The Institute will be affiliated with the University of the West Indies and the University of Guyana, and students from abroad will be admitted.

The Government has indicated that it does not expect to engender a utopia, but in the proposals listed, as compared to the great waste of manpower and material in the past system, it is expected that the average Guyanese will take pride in the new health services and in their smooth running. Overall, it is hoped that with these new methods of treatment there will be a large decrease of the work days wasted in seeking out medical care and attention.

Summary

Hospitals were started in Guyana in the eighteenth century. The military hospitals were organized in the nineteenth century and eventually became colonial hospitals. The conditions in these hospitals were abominable. In the year 1844, 300 beds were provided for the colonial hospitals and general hospitals, and an out-patient department was started. The credit for the medical and public health development in Guyana goes to Dr. George Giglioli, who laid the foundation for the eradication of malaria by means of a very skillfully designed scheme of house-spraying with DDT. The existing medical structure concentrates on both the curative and preventive aspects of medicine. The dispensaries, public hospitals, and district cottage hospitals practice curative medicine. Preventive medicine includes all aspects of work done on environmental sanitation and in the training of health care professionals in providing adequate nutrition for the nation.

3

Public Health Services

Prior to independence, Guyana had a very poor record for providing public health services; however, with recent improvements in public health facilities, such as a pure water supply, adequate sanitation, and the impact of DDT in the control of malaria, the country has moved in the direction of improved health care services for its citizens. The improved health conditions are reflected in the steady decline of infant and general mortality rates over the past thirty or forty years.

Health Services Before Independence

The hospitals of the country were administered by the government medical department. There were five government general hospitals and three specialty hospitals for the treatment of leprosy, tuberculosis, and mental illness. Hospitals with limited facilities were also established on individual estates by the B. G. Sugar Producers' Association. A medical clinic was also located on each estate which was visited by a physician at regular intervals.

The medical department had a staff of fifty to sixty full-time and part-time medical officers, including specialists and local health officers. Over the years, prior to independence, there had been great difficulty in filling the specialists' positions due to the inadequate salaries offered to qualified candidates.

In 1957, there were 125 medical officers practicing in the country, of whom 66 were employed by the government. There were 23 dentists in private practice and four in government service.

Public health services were indeed limited by the number of health care practitioners. In many cases, there was immense dissatisfaction among physicians due to the poor equipment, depressing wards, long working hours, and lack of recognition for younger doctors who did not get the cooperation and guidance of senior physicians. The hospital administrator suggested that a strong medical board was needed to hire and fire health care professionals who did not adequately carry out their duties, but the problem was compounded by the principle of supply and demand. If the supply were large, then the necessary disciplining of doctors could have taken place without serious consequences to patients.

One hospital administrator noted that several physicians usually took "leave of absence" during the Christmas holidays—a period during which their services were most needed. Doctors took unfair advantage of the staffing situation and passed this habit on to the younger physicians, resulting in a vicious cycle perpetuating the ineffective delivery of health care services to the public. We shall now turn our attention to various programs instituted over the years in the area of public health.

Development and Future of the Malaria Eradication Campaign

Since Dr. Giglioli had done so much valuable work in the area of malaria eradication, we again present his further views as they were given on Radio Demerara. Dr. Giglioli stated:

> During 1945 and 1946, experiments with DDT were carried out on a progressively increasing scale. We also perfected our techniques; we found that a single application of DDT to a group of ranges on Lusignan Estate continued to kill the mosquito carriers of both malaria and yellow fever for over two years. DDT durability was not as spectacular in houses of a better type; its duration was proportionate to the degree of sophistication of the tenants; the greater the tendency to resist spraying operations, and to wipe the insecticide off the walls and furniture even before the spraying teams had left the premises. These studies enabled us to lengthen the intervals between sprayings, from 6 to 12 and finally to 18 months, with great reduction in costs.
>
> Meanwhile malaria transmission was controlled on both the Demerara and Berbice estuaries, 60,000 persons being protected directly by house spraying and the residents of Georgetown being protected indirectly by the control of malaria in the surrounding area.
>
> In January 1947, the Malaria Research and Yellow Fever Services merged, and a systematic countrywide attack on *Anopheles darlingi* and *Aedes Aegypti* was begun.
>
> In the same year, operations were extended to the far interior; Dr. Ramjattan and I toured the Rupununi District, surveying the malaria situation, and ourselves spraying with DDT a number of villages on Savannahs. We had no sooner returned from this trip when a severe outbreak of fever was reported among the Patamana Indians. Colonel Gunn, the Commander of the American Base at Atkinson Field, flew me in on a small plane; we landed on a tiny and very uneven strip on the top of a mountain between the upper Potaro and the Ireng Rivers. At the late Mr. Tesserick's diamond workings at Valgrad, I saw many

Indians with malaria, and discovered *Anopheles darlingi* in the house, and its larva in the flooded diamond gravel pits close to the camp.

Just seven days later, two spraying teams flew to Orinduik on the Ireng River. One team, headed by Dr. Ramjattan and Colonel G. Moorhead, then Commissioner of Lands and Mines, toured the northern part of the area, with Mr. Tesserick as guide and the late Father Keary, S. J., as interpreter. Mr. Hamid Mohamen and I, with Mr. Albert Brazao as our guide, took the southern sector. When our parties separated, the leaders of my group took the wrong trail, and for the next nine days my companions and I lived on a strict diet of rice and condensed milk, which we had with us for distribution to the Indians. Though monotonous, this diet supplied all the energy required for scrambling up and down those tough, steep mountains for 7 or 8 hours a day. Vitamins were supplied by the large calabashes of Kasheerie supplied by the Patamonas. These were very welcome, refreshing and invigorating when on the march or during spraying operations.

The feelings were somewhat different in the chilly hours after dawn, when we were busy breaking up camp to proceed on our way, when the Tushawa appeared with a large valedictory calabash of cold, livid fluid; good manners, however, required us to take a long drink and show appreciation.

At the end of nine days, the two parties rendezvoused at Orinduik having sprayed every known house and camp within this very impervious area. That was the last of malaria among the Patamonas; subsequent surveys have shown no trace of it.

In 1948, all the coastlands and lower rivers districts had been sprayed repeatedly. In a comprehensive report published in August of 1948, I was able to make the following statement:

All the evidence available indicates the *Anopheles darlingi* (the local carrier of malaria) and *Aedes Aegypti* (the vector of yellow fever) have been eradicated from the treated areas, some 200 miles of coastlands and estuary banks.

In a foreword to my report, Dr. Fred L. Soper, the Director of the Pan American Health Organization, wrote as follows:

The initial work with DDT in British Guiana began at a time when the use of insecticide was restricted almost entirely to military operations. Fortunately, the careful entomological and parasitological studies inaugurated in the colony some years before the introduction of DDT have been continued; these give a basis for comparison with results obtained under difficult conditions in a highly malarial region in the tropics, and should be an important factor in furthering the organization of nationwide programs elsewhere.

The World Health Organization has been mainly responsible for the development of malaria eradication campaigns throughout the world. This great organization, however, was founded in 1948, the same year in which, in Guyana, we had already published a report on the eradication of malaria and its carrier from our coastlands by the new DDT technique.

It was Dr. Soper who inspired and pioneered the grandiose concept of worldwide malaria eradication, which was accepted by the Americans in 1954 at the XIV Pan American Sanitary Conference held in Mexico City, under Soper's chairmanship. In 1955, the VIIIth World Health Assembly in Geneva passed a resolution to "implement a program having as its ultimate objective, the worldwide eradication of malaria". The data collected in Guyana, between 1945 and 1948, and published in 1948, supplied the earliest and best documented information on the practical possibility of malaria eradication by the new DDT technique, and as such, paved the way for the most ambitious public health program ever conceived—the world-wide eradication of malaria.

In the sparsely inhabited, remote interior, *Anopheles darlingi* could not survive by feeding on man exclusively, as it did on the densely populated coastlands; it feeds on animals as well as man, and lives in the forest where malaria transmission may thus take place.

Indians pass much of their existence in the forest cultivating their farms, hunting, fishing and bleeding balata [a rubberlike gum from the bully tree]. Within the forest, DDT is of little use, as there are no proper houses for spraying.

International frontiers constitute another problem in the interior, as they are not respected by either the *Anopheles* or the malaria parasites. Full results cannot be achieved without effective international collaboration.

For these reasons, malaria had continued to occur in more remote parts of the interior, in spite of the fact that it had disappeared from the coastlands and lower river districts where nine-tenths of our population live, free from the disease.

With the elimination of the mosquito carrier, the arrival of persons infected with malaria within the coastal area caused little concern, as the opportunity of transmission was not there. We were badly jolted, however, in 1961; a sudden discovery was made of a number of cases of *benigne tertian* malaria on both the East and West banks of the Demerara estuary.

In all, we identified 108 cases, but no *Anopheles darlingi* could be found. We discovered instead that another mosquito, known by the name of *Anopheles aquasalis* was to blame. This is a very common mosquito all along our coast where it favors salt and brackish waters for breeding. Our investigations between 1934 and 1948 had shown that it had a distinct preference for the blood of livestock and animals, and that it did not enter houses and did not attack man with that insistence and repetition which are necessary for malaria transmission. The progressive reduction of the livestock population on the Demerara estuary, due to lack of pastures taken over by housing and by industrial developments, and by rice cultivation and even more so, to the ever-increasing mechanization on the roads and in the fields, have caused *Anopheles aquasalis* to turn to man for its blood meals; it thus became an active malaria transmitter as soon as the infection was brought to the area by persons who had contracted the disease in the Northwest District. This malaria outbreak signaled a new and very real danger, as the changes which have occurred on the Demerara estuary are only an example of a general trend throughout the coastlands.

For this reason, the eradication of malaria from the remote interior, and a tighter surveillance on travelers became an urgent necessity.

In the interior, we introduced an entirely new technique developed in Brazil, but never previously tested on an adequate scale and under strict administrative and scientific control. This technique did not aim against the mosquito; it consists of incorporating an anti-malarial drug in the general supply of kitchen salt. The aim is to suppress malaria infestation in the population. The Chloroquinized Salt Campaign was inaugurated in January 1961 and concluded in December 1965. It was carried out with the financial and technical assistance of the World Health Organization, the American Health Organization, and UNICEF. Even with this technique, difficulties have been encountered. In the Rupununi, the campaign was handicapped by the smuggling of ordinary salt from Brazil, and in 1962 a new strain of malaria parasite was introduced from across the border, which was resistant to chloroquine, and thus was not suppressed by the medicated salt; a return to DDT was necessary. In some very inaccessible localities, where there are no shops and the local Indian population is poor, the medicated salt did not reach people regularly in a sufficient quantity. This happened on the upper Barima River, where a flareup of *benigne tertian* malaria, extending to the upper Barima and Kaituma River, has been recorded during the past three months.

From Venezuela, we have reports of some cases on the Guyuni and Wenamu frontier, another extremely inaccessible area.

Apart from these very recent developments which have as yet not been fully evaluated but constitute a serious setback, the general malaria situation in Guyana can be gauged by the returns for the year 1965, during which blood samples were taken by field and laboratory personnel of the Malaria Eradication Services of the Ministry of Health, from 61,242 persons. In 1965, the country's population was estimated at 640,000. There was no malaria recorded from coastlands and near interior; none from the Northwest, the Guyuni, the Mazaruni and Potaro districts, and from the Pakaraima Plateau and the North Rupununi Savannah. There were 22 positive cases in the South Rupununi Savannah, all from an area of less than ten square miles. There was a single isolated case from Orealla on the Corentyne, which probably originated in Surinam. That makes a total of twenty-three cases in all out of a population of 640,000 and 61,242 persons specifically examined. Up to 1945, this same number of cases could have been diagnosed at any time among the children in any one school between Morawahanna and the Canje River.

It has been said that Guyana has a continental destiny; malariaologically speaking, this is a fact and not a theory. All our neighbors have malaria problems which are not likely to be solved in the foreseeable future. With hard work and perseverance, we may succeed in attaining eradication on a nationwide basis. That would be great, in fact, a unique achievement for a tropical, continent country. Even so, I see no prospect for our ever being able to disarm and rest on our laurels; an efficient, permanent and properly directed malaria laboratory and field service are essential in our public health organization, if we are not to wake up some dark morning to find ourselves on the high road back to our starting point. It should also be remembered that if *Anopheles aquasalis* became the malaria transmitter as it was in 1961 on the Demerara estuary, control would be infinitely more difficult and more expensive.

In the same year, Dr. Giglioli gave a very remarkable history of how DDT came to Guyana:

> I will begin this broadcast with a quotation from a paper written in 1919 by Dr. K.S. Wise, then Surgeon General of British Guiana. Dr. Wise was a far better writer than I am, and I feel that I cannot improve on his words in order to convey to the Guyanese of today, what malaria in the past meant to this country. I quote:
>
> "Malaria is the pivot on which most of our problems of public health balance; its basal influence is the substratum from which our difficulties arise.
>
> "This is not an exaggeration. Malaria is as omnipresent as the light and wind, a blight on our land checking and distorting the growth of the community. Bathed in malaria and saturated with its poison, the people are handicapped at birth, live an infancy and childhood with a millstone round their necks while those who survive resent an influence they do not understand.

"The enormous loss of individual efficiency, the steadily recurring loss of prosperity in a people afflicted in this way, the subnormal character of physical education and normal life under the above circumstances is obvious enough.

"The colony staggers under a series of vicious cycles which at present show no surcease. Malaria steadily increases the demand for expenditure, for relief, while diminishing the power to supply revenue; increases its own license for damage while diminishing the power to resist. Malaria has indeed stolen the life of this country. It has intimately woven its fatal thread through almost each and every pattern of our life and thus it stalks an always menacing figure throughout the length and breadth of the land."

What Dr. Wise wrote in 1919, was still fully valid in 1944, when under Governor Sir Gordon Lethem, a number of extensive land reclamation schemes throughout the coastland were drafted and given very considerable publicity. To this layman, such schemes brought promise of agricultural expansion, greater employment, greater production and prosperity; to the malariaologist, familiar with the local problem, they spelled inexorably an expansion of endemic malaria to healthy coastal areas such as the Corentyne, which were at the time relatively free from the disease, and the main source of increment in the Colony's population.

The tragedy of malaria in this country was its marriage to agricultural development, for the simple reason that the same factors such as sea defenses, drainage and irrigation, which made agriculture possible in the coastlands, also transformed them into ideal, permanent, all-season breeding grounds for one of the world's most dangerous malaria carrying mosquitos, known to science as *Anopheles darlingi*. In all the coastal areas best organized for agriculture, from the Essequibo Coast to the Berbice Estuary, malaria prevailed, and the progress of the population was stagnant as births, as an average, barely balanced deaths, and in some years there was an excess of deaths over births.

The population of Guyana developed from wave after wave of immigrants from distant lands, brought to the country to work on its plantations. There, they were made to live, and malaria became a habit, a way of life, as they knew no other. They developed no knowledge or tradition in respect to its avoidance as is found, for instance, in the ancient malaria countries of the Mediterranean.

The true nature of the disease was generally misunderstood; the fever frequently manifested itself with slight jaundice, bilious vomiting, dark colored urine and bilious diarrhea; surely this was only "biliousness", and the proper treatment was a good purge. This was Hippocratic medicine at its best, but 25 centuries out of date! I think this country in the not too distant past, used to import nearly as many tons of purgatives as it exported tons of sugar! Quinine was taken as a last resort and usually in insufficient doses, and for too short a period.

Malaria frequently caused abortion and miscarriage, yet there was a deeply entrenched prejudice against quinine in this respect; many expectant mothers lost their babies through deliberate avoidance of the one drug that would have saved them.

The problem was immense, and aggravated by ignorance and prejudice. Yet in the turn of only five years, between 1945 and 1950, malaria disappeared from the coastlands and the near interior, and became rare even in the more remote districts.

How did this miracle take place? DDT did it; of that there is no doubt, but was that all? Not entirely; other factors, and a great deal of good luck intervened to bring the new insecticide to render its proper application, immediate, economic and efficient, at a time when knowledge on this entirely new technique was scanty and practically unobtainable.

DDT was discovered as far back as 1876; for close to 60 years its properties remained unknown. In 1938, it was found to be useful as an agricultural insecticide. When the Japanese entered the War in 1941, the main source of pyrethrum was lost to the allied armies. This was the most effective insecticide at that time used for the control of body lice and the prevention of typhus fever, the great pestilence of warring armies. A frantic search for pyrethrum substitutes then started, and thousands of chemicals, new and old, were screened for this purpose, among them, DDT. It was found that it remained active for weeks and even months if it was sprayed on walls or clothing. The sprayed surfaces remained lethal to all insects that alighted on them. No previously known insecticide had had such revolutionary properties.

The experimental development of DDT research, its large-scale manufacture, the results of trials in the field, and in the course of military operations, all took place under strict war secrecy. In the malaria infested jungles of Burma, the allied troops advanced under its protection, while the Japanese suffered innumerable casualties from malaria. In Naples just after its occupation, typhus fever exploded; it was nipped in the bud by DDT. All this, however, proceeded under the veil of secrecy, and not a single report of DDT appeared in the scientific press.

Let us now return to the land reclamation schemes which were being drafted and publicized in Guyana in 1944. As I have said, in the light of malariaological knowledge then available, these schemes carried grave malaria implications. As Government Malariaologist at that time, I made the necessary representations, but with no effect. Dr. Heatherington, the D.M.S., and I then called on Mr. Heap, the Colonial Secretary, to explain the problem. Mr. Heap quickly grasped the situation, but even so, no practical progress was made until a remarkable chain of lucky events not only offered us the break we needed, but also far more than we had ever expected or hoped for.

In July 1944, Mr. Heap was Officer Administering the Government, in the absence of Sir Gordon Lethem, then on leave. On the 13th of that month, three very important persons turned up in Georgetown quite unexpectedly; they were Sir Robert Robinson, the President of the Royal Society, Sir John Simondson, F.R.S., and Dr. Alexander King. The first two were the chairman and a member, respectively, of the Board which, during the War, was responsible for the control and the allocation of chemicals, explosives and insecticides. Dr. King resided in Washington and provided the exchange of scientific information between Washington and London. These scientists were traveling from Washington on war business. Their plane developed trouble and was held up in Trinidad for three days; they took this opportunity for a quick, unofficial and entirely unscheduled flight to Georgetown.

In the course of general conversation at the Government House on the progress of the war, the major contribution of DDT to the Burma Campaign was mentioned. Mr. Heap was immediately interested, and he brought up our own grave malaria predicament in relation to the proposed land reclamation schemes. To his everlasting credit, Mr. Heap grasped this unusual and totally unexpected opportunity to arrange a conference at the Government House, on the following morning, for a more thorough discussion. At this conference, I outlined the malaria situation, and the inevitable connection between agricultural development and the spread and intensification of malaria. Dr. King described the new properties of DDT and the experimental field trials made in the U.S.A. and in West Africa, and the practical results achieved in the various tropical war theatres.

From that very moment, much of the knowledge we had patiently accumulated over the past 20 years, suddenly ceased to be of purely academic interest, and became basic information for the practical control of malaria.

From our studies at Blairmont, later extended to all other sugar estates, we knew, in fact, that malaria in Guyana was transmitted by a single species, *anopheles darlingi*, this mosquito having a specific preference for human blood. It attacked inside the houses, on which it converged from its far flung breeding places, and after gorging itself with human blood, it rested for many hours within the houses, on the walls and furnishings.

Henceforth, our antimalaria battlefield would be in the human habitation; we could forget surface waters. The prospects for malaria control so dismal only a few minutes previous, suddenly appeared bright and promising.

What Dr. King told us was so new and unexpected, that at the time, it sounded rather like a fairy tale. I was able, however, to inform the meeting that in *Anopheles darlingi* in British Guiana, we had the ideal mosquito for DDT. I can remember using the words "a mosquito made to order for DDT." From the general discussion that followed, our distinguished visitors were adequately convinced and before the meeting broke up, a cable was dispatched to London releasing half a ton of DDT for experimental work in this country.

The entry in my diary for the 14th of July, 1944, though laconic, made interesting reading: "Conference at the Government House on DDT—Went home with fever; blood positive for malaria parasites." We can thus say that the malaria parasite itself sat in at the conference which marked its undoing.

In January, 1945, half a ton of DDT arrived in this country and with it some spraying equipment loaned from the U.S. Department of Agriculture. Messrs. Symes and Hadaway, both entomologists, came out to help us during the first three months of our work. We had no literature or reports on the use of DDT, only some rather approximate information on the preparation of solutions for spraying, and the dosage to be applied. Everything had to be worked out and organized from scratch. On the malaria situation, on the contrary, both as regards the distribution and incidence of the disease and of its Anophiline carrier, we had full statistical records going several years back, covering both the coastlines and interior. Within a week we were able to begin spraying operations at Lusignan and Mon Repos, and a little later in Lodge Village.

In military practice, up to that time, DDT had been used lavishly, expense being no object under war conditions; it was broadcast from airplanes, it was sprayed in camps and houses, it was applied to surface waters; aerosol bombs were also first invented so that the soldiers might protect themselves in their fox-holes.

In the country, we had the knowledge to use DDT intelligently and economically; we applied DDT where it would hurt the most, to the interior of houses exclusively—and every house in the country was eventually sprayed. The techniques we developed in the last few months have not been changed since, and we would not change them if the whole campaign had to be repeated today.[1]

This extended quotation of Dr. Giglioli's analysis of the malaria eradication brings us up to the present. We will now focus attention on other areas of public health services in Guyana.

Current Public Health Services

The discussion of current public health service may be divided into three sub-topics: 1) environmental cleanliness; 2) indigenous herb cures and local efforts; and 3) children and health care.

Environmental Cleanliness

A clean environment obviates many health problems. Since Georgetown is below high tide level, the city faces two serious problems: 1) it has to be protected from the sea and 2) the excess water has to be drained off during the rainy season. With assistance from the central government, the Georgetown City Council has constructed a large scale drainage system using high powered electrical pumps. The traditional gravitational drainage system has been converted into a mechanical operation which is now functioning smoothly and effectively. To make this system more efficient, all the main canals have been deepened by the continued use of the Hymac machine. There is widespread concern that this development may create new ecological problems due to the dredging operation creating large deposits of silt exposed to the forces of erosion.

The Mayor and the Georgetown City Council have made great efforts to provide a clean neighborhood. To avoid infection of edibles the Mayor has given the following directions:

1. Bearded males are asked to wear clean beard coverings.
2. Employees who handle food must not smoke or chew tobacco, at least not while they handle food.
3. Persons with communicable diseases should not be allowed on any part of the food premises.
4. Persons with an open injury, sores, or other lesions on exposed parts of the body shall not be allowed in food handling areas.
5. All eating houses should be clean, free from nuisances and contamination.

Meat dealers and butchers were given similar direction. In trying to judge the quality of meat, the following precautions can be kept in mind: 1) color of the meat is a good indicator of the condition of the meat —pinkish or pale red meat being a sign of high quality, 2) dark red fibres often are signs of coarse meat, and 3) flabby and sticky meat should never be offered for sale in the market. Both buyer and seller must make every effort to maintain a high standard of hygiene in the meat selling process.

The stallholders have created health and sanitation problems in Georgetown. The Mayor passed an ordinance aimed at correcting health and sanitation problems in Georgetown, but the vendors failed to cooperate with these efforts. The fish and shrimp vendors who continued to create health hazards were ordered by the Mayor to evacuate their stalls.

The Jamaican Food and Nutrition Institute (JFNI) held a week-long conference at the Tower Hotel focusing on discussions aimed at developing methods of improving foods for babies after weaning. The conference concentrated on three specific areas: 1) the problem of protein malnutrition, 2) mothers discontinuing breast feeding, 3) misleading advertisements by the news media.

In light of these persistent problems, the seminar concentrated on improvement of eating habits and proper growing and distribution of goods. The seminar devised plans for proper eating habits, and the government is well disposed toward these plans. The Caribbean countries were willing to implement them as a comprehensive health care system for a developing nation. The Mayor reminded the people about environmental cleanliness through his weekly broadcasting and he warned the vendors in particular to keep the city clean.

The members of the International Society for Krishna Consciousness provide an example of cleanliness of environments where food is served. They are punctilious about two things, namely, peace and cleanliness. The Hindus, particularly the Brahmans, have a great sense of cleanliness. The cook must bathe and put on new clothes before entering the kitchen. As he cooks he should never touch his mouth and no one should taste or test the food before it is offered to Krishna. There is a spiritual element to food.

Indigenous Herb Cures and Local Efforts

In Guyana, the dispensing of good medical care is often limited or compromised by the unavailability of many drugs, equipment and other necessities elsewhere associated with the practice of modern medicine. This has in no small way discouraged young Guyanese physicians and surgeons who have been recently trained abroad from returning to their homeland.

Guyana, like almost all new developing countries whose economy is not supported by oil, suffers a severe shortage in hard currency for trade in the international market. Guyana's commercial exports are substantially outbalanced by its import of essential supplies. This, of course, leads to inevitable embargoes by government regulations and controls. To reduce the occasional shortage of essential drugs, the government is trying to manufacture some of them locally. This has improved the situation significantly, but not enough to answer fully local demands.

Because of their background, Guyanese in nearly all walks of life still demonstrate a strong belief in local herb medicines. The government has been undertaking research into these areas to determine whether they have valid curative properties that can be confirmed by scientific investigations.

Drugs are usually adequate in Guyana, but they are expensive. Since there are still some diseases which are cured by herbs, the Guyana government is encouraging a group of doctors and other professionals to establish "The International College of Naturopathy and Applied Science." This institute experiments with medical herbs to produce drugs intended to cure syphilis, cancer and other diseases. The Institute will be affiliated with the University of the West Indies and the University of Guyana. There is also another research center at Katobo which is trying to produce a chemical from termite secretion to cure cancer.

While it has long been known that alcohol causes cirrhosis of the liver, it has lately been discovered by doctors that bush tea has also been a contributing factor. Researchers in Guyana have to infer the cause of cirrhosis from the rates reported from other countries, as in North America, India, Africa, and Japan. These countries caution their people not to consume *Senecio Crotalaria Fulva* (bush tea) alkaloids because they cause hepatitis and cirrhosis of the liver. Guyanese chemists must continue to carry on research in this area as it is well known that care must be taken not to depend too much on research from other countries because of different and varying conditions. Research is being done in crystal venom from the muscle, which is presently used for neuromuscular disorders and cancer.

According to local belief, leaves from pumpkin, sweet potato, cassava, watercress, tamarind, and lettuce, as well as banana flower buds, have medicinal effects when consumed raw. (These leaves contain protein and vitamins.)

The people contribute much toward national health care and donate their labor. Two medical centers have recently been built, one in Karaudaunawa and the other at Shew. In addition, a substantial amount of funds has been provided by the government of Guyana and by U.S. AID (Agency for International Development). Each of the centers at present provides medical care for about 620 persons.

With money and materials provided by the government and through the U.S. AID Program, Guyana has entered into a medical self-help program, resulting in the opening of a Medical Hut in Awarewanau at a cost of $7,000. At Aishalton, the Amerindian Girls' Hotel was built with people contributing their labor, to accommodate female trainee health workers. The Community Health Workers Training Program is sponsored jointly by the Inter-American Development Bank and the Government of Guyana.

The Jaycees of Georgetown published a 40-page booklet (now in its second edition) entitled "Be Brite . . . Eat Right." The purpose of this publication is to generate and support programs aimed at the continued use of indigenous foods in order to provide greater self-sufficiency in the country. A new section dealing with infant nutrition and snacks for school children is a recent addition to the book. Dr. B. E. C. Hopwood, Health and Manpower Consultant from the Commonwealth Secretariat, held discussions with the Caribbean Territory Health authorities. Dr. Hopwood sought a grant from AID to be used for training personnel in health-related fields. He also expressed his great appreciation for the efforts that had been made to eradicate malaria from Guyana, while at the same time encouraging the health officials never to relax their efforts in continuing the work to eliminate the unhealthy conditions found in Caribbean countries and in Guyana. Regional health officers with specialized training in diabetes and hypertension have been requested.

Children and Health Care

Mothers are warned of the dangers of keeping a dirty home. They are told that not only does this condition attract disease-bearing flies and vermin, but small infants crawling on filthy floors almost always acquire intestinal parasites such as worms.

Infant immunization is a compulsory feature of the country's health program. It has long been so, even before independence. Parents are required to produce evidence in the form of a certificate that their children have been immunized.

When a baby is two weeks old it is given BCG to protect it from tuberculosis. Later, when the baby is twelve weeks old, OPV and DPT are administered. The child is fully immunized against most childhood diseases before entering nursery school. Children are given dental health care as well. Injections of measles and influenza vaccines, however, are not compulsory in Guyana.

Summary

Since its independence the country has made encouraging progress in attempting to control endemic and, at times, even epidemic diseases.

The government of independent Guyana is, of course, more sensitive and attentive to the problems and needs of its people than when, as a colony, decisive power resided at Whitehall in London.

Programs in health education are vigorously pushed. Every effort is made to create positive attitudes toward sanitation and cleanliness. The health value of well balanced meals is continually stressed. Government also encourages scientific research on the many local herbs, which for generations have been used as folk medicines by the people. Previously, the use of these herbs has been recommended only by folklore and superstition. This new respect for the past engenders acceptance of modern medical advances.

Finally, the vigorous implementation of the immunization laws is already being reflected in a significant drop in the statistics of infant and childhood morbidity and mortality.

4

Health Education in Guyana

History of Education

During the period of slavery, planters objected to the education of blacks. In 1738, Hermanus Post brought two Moravian Brethren to Berbice in the northeastern section of Guyana, to a mission for the Amerindians, 100 miles upriver, in order to prevent the black slaves from being disturbed by the teachings of Christianity. The colonial government officially opposed admitting to the colony any missionaries who might establish schools for the slaves; therefore, the colony was divided into twelve parishes—seven Anglican and five Church of Scotland. In that way, it was felt that the activities of missionaries could be controlled.

Meanwhile, there was a growing population of mulattoes. These children, whose fathers were white, were given preference over all but the so-called "pure white." By 1800, there was evidence of an effort to separate ethnic groups in the several schools. One school, located at Stabroek, was for boys and girls under the direction of Elizabeth Goddard. Around 1827, a school was opened for "free boys," and later, one for "free girls" of "all complexions." The colonial governor, Sir Benjamin d'Urban, was active in the establishment of this school. Each subscriber paid a fee of thirty gilders (about six U.S. dollars), which entitled the subscriber to nominate one child for free admission to the school.

In 1833, the Emancipation Act was passed. Included in this act was a provision for the education of blacks. Under this new spirit, the government began to invite missionaries of various religious groups to Guyana to establish churches and schools. In December of 1835, the first grant (US $4,800) for Negro education in British Guiana was made by the British government. By 1841, there were 101 denominational schools in the country.[1]

In 1852, George Denis was named the first Inspector of Schools. One of the central issues at that time was whether church groups should continue to control schools or whether all schools should be brought under secular control. Denis favored secular control; however, given the condition of education in England at that time, a strong, centralized, government-controlled system of education could not be imposed on a missionary colony like British Guiana.

One of the major problems confronting education was the insufficiency of well-trained teachers, which Mr. Denis noted in his report of 1833. The colony's government had proposed a teachers' training college as early as 1836. In 1851, the Anglicans established Bishop's College to train theological students and announced the establishment of a Normal Seminary for teachers of the Church of England.

Oral teacher examinations began in 1853 to certify the ability to read accurately, to write clearly and easily, to spell correctly, and to do arithmetic problems using the four fundamental rules of addition, subtraction, division, and multiplication. Those who had a practical knowledge of educational principles received an additional salary of $100 per year. Written examinations were begun in 1854, and in 1855 these examinations were divided into three "grades" so that a teacher was designated as either first, second, or third class. Remnants of this classification system still remained when Guyana became independent. Third class teachers could read accurately and fluently, write easily and legibly, spell correctly, work mathematical problems using the four rules, and point out the parts of speech in a simple sentence. A second class teacher was able to read easily and intelligently with expression and correct pronunciation, to write and spell correctly, to understand the rules for instruction in writing, to add, subtract, multiply, divide, work proportion problems, understand weights and measures and understand the general outline of history and geography. A first class teacher was expected to possess all these abilities in addition to being able to do mental arithmetic, and to demonstrate a knowledge of natural philosophy and history, bookkeeping, and the First Book of *Euclid*. Women teachers were expected to know needlework and music but were excused from geometry and bookkeeping.[2]

By the Education Ordinance of 1855, schools were owned or operated by Christian denominations and the government agreed to maintain school buildings and pay teachers' salaries. This meant that all schools were bound to a system of dual control, a policy that was not effectively changed until independence.[3]

A compulsory education law was passed in 1876. In general, school attendance remained rather poor because child labor represented a valuable source of family income. The East Indians who lived on the sugar estates were particularly reluctant to have their children attend school. During the earliest years of their settlement, their major objective was to acquire wealth. In many instances, everything was sacrificed to achieve this goal, and it was not unusual for the estate Indians to combine their family's wealth, convert it to gold and diamonds, then bury or hide the family fortune. When these families gained some wealth (although often their wealth was deliberately not made public), sons would be sent to school so that they could enter the professions. The educated sons never returned to the estates; they stayed in Georgetown and manipulated the family money to create highly lucrative businesses and to arrange affluent marriages for their sisters and daughters. Black families sought education and westernization as a means of social advancement. However, in many instances, lacking substantial finances, black families' fortunes tended to rise and fall on individual ability rather than to maintain a steady societal position. In general, Indian girls were not allowed to attend school because families were afraid that education would prevent their contracting a suitable marriage. Black daughters were more likely to obtain a formal education than their Indian counterparts, although they still did not have the same opportunity for education that the boys had. Given these societal conditions, it is not surprising that the school attendance rate for the Indian population was only one per cent in 1890 and 50 per cent in 1921.

The system of education that evolved in Guyana during its colonial period was in many ways similar to the educational system of England. Primary education was organized through denominational groups or proprietary schools with the government maintaining the schools and paying the teachers. Children had to purchase their own books and supplies; if families failed to do this, then the child had to manage as well as possible without school materials. At the age of eleven, children completed primary school. At this point a child's future education was largely determined by family wealth and position or by innate ability. Each of the three counties had a scholarship and the winners were assured a place in the government secondary school—Queen's for boys and Bishop's for girls.

Those who were poor but hoped to break the poverty cycle would take the School Leaving Certificate Examination. If successful, they could become apprenticed as teachers or enter the Teachers' Training Institute. During their training as teacher, or subsequent to their training, some of these students would attempt the examinations given to secondary school students. All secondary schools except Queen's and Bishop's were denominational, and every secondary school, including the two government schools, had a fee requirement. The government secondary schools and two Catholic Schools—St. Stanislaus, established by the Jesuits in 1866, and the Convent of the Sacred Heart run by the Ursulines—were considered the most prestigious. The better the reputation of the secondary school, the higher the fees. Schools at the "top" of the ladder usually gave a qualifying examination for entrance in order to keep classes small. Very often, however, family influence overcame test results.

Once in secondary school, all students took courses directed toward successful standing in the Junior Cambridge School Certificate Examination. The Senior Cambridge was usually taken during the last year of secondary school when a student was about eighteen. However, as there were many proprietary secondary schools, older students or young teachers often "sat the examinations" as registered students of these schools in addition to students actually completing their secondary school education.

The Cambridge Examinations were external examinations, graded in England and taken by all colonial students as well as by those attending school in England. One could pass Senior Cambridge at the first, second, or third class level. Of greater significance, however, was the combination of grades that one received in each subject. A proper combination of credits and distinctions would give a student the distinction of receiving the London Matriculation Certificate. That certificate was necessary for entrance to any university in England. Students who passed the school Certificate Examination, but failed to get the Matriculation, had to pass another examination. In the late 1950s the system was replaced by the Ordinary and Advanced Level Examinations which are still being used in England.

Thus, prior to independence, education was largely geared to the educational traditions of England. This gave a marked advantage to those who were wealthy, but even among the wealthy, admission to a university was a most difficult achievement. Although technical education was available, it was sporadic, insufficient and lacked social prestige in a country where social appearances were of great consequence.[4]

Current Educational Development

Some educational reforms were begun prior to Guyana's independence from England. These were important steps toward educational autonomy, providing opportunities for students unable to travel to England, India or the United States to receive advanced education. Students of good ability but poor circumstances can now, without much difficulty, complete their secondary education.

Once independence had been achieved, the government recognized as its first great challenge the reconciling and unifying of the various ethnic and social groups, still sharply divided and at times overtly hostile to each other. It recognized as a priority the elimination of conditions which fostered intergroup antagonism and the development of a social, political, and economic climate in which the aspirations of all groups could find satisfying fulfillment. This meant assuring equality of opportunities, including equal academic and technical training available to all.

In order to bring this about, the government began by abolishing all private schools. Schools which had been run by religious orders became a part of the government program. All students were to be trained in the same curriculum, under conditions which were to be as similar as possible. This focus attempted to give meaning to the national ideology expressed in the motto, "One People, One Nation, One Destiny."

Further, the government enacted the National Service Act, making it compulsory for all youth to serve in the National Service Corps for a period of at least two years. Unlike the drafting of youth in other countries, the Guyana Youth Corps is not oriented toward military preparedness. The emphasis is to educate the young in technical training to enable them to use their own developed skills in developing the national resources of their country.

The present educational system has children enter nursery school at the age of three years nine months and stay until the age of five years nine months. At this stage, education is considered to be informal and primarily concerned with teaching the child to get along with others and to develop a good attitude toward education. The child enters primary school at approximately six years of age and remains until the age of eleven. Following primary school, a child takes the Secondary School Entrance Examination. Children are allowed to take this examination from the age of nine to eleven, depending upon their ability. It is important to note that this examination is prepared in Guyana and graded by Guyanese educational professionals.

The results of the examination determine the type of secondary school that the child is permitted to enter. The new Multilateral Secondary School is similar to the traditional secondary school. St. Stanislaus College has already been converted into a Multilateral School; Queen's, Bishop's, St. Joseph's, and the Convent of the Sacred Heart are moving toward the Multilateral school curriculum, which is somewhat more comprehensive than the schools' previous curriculum. The Multilateral school program takes five years to complete, and the conversion to its program was expected to be achieved in the early 1980s.[5]

Students who do not do well on the Secondary School Entrance Examination go to Community High Schools. After three years at the Community High School, the student takes Part I of the Secondary School Proficiency Examination. If the student does well on this examination, he is transferred to a Multilateral School. If he does not, he continues at the Community High School for another year. During that year the student takes part in a work study program of vocational education. At the end of this fourth year of study, the student takes Part II of the Secondary School Proficiency Examination. Students who complete the Community High School program are awarded a Secondary School Proficiency Diploma.[6]

Part I of the Secondary School Proficiency test consists of papers in mathematics, English language, social studies, general reasoning and science. Part II of the Secondary School Proficiency test is a paper on the theory and practice of the vocation the student has chosen. The student may select one or two "vocations" depending on the school that the child attends. On a country-wide basis, vocational training programs are available in agricultural science, tailoring, home economics, crafts, motor mechanics, electronics, electrical installation, carpentry, welding, and music/drama/dance.

Students at the Multilateral schools also receive special technical training. During the first and second years, the curriculum at the Multilateral School includes art, crafts, and home economics. During the third year, students are required to take either industrial arts or home economics. At the end of the third year these students enter one of two streams—Technical A, for those more gifted academically, or Technical B, for those more practically oriented. Those who complete Technical A can earn a certificate "equivalent" to the Ordinary Level of the School Certificate. The Technical A students also have an opportunity to enter the University of Guyana under the Faculty of Technology or the Technical Institutes for technical courses. The Technical Institutes' craft courses are open to those who complete Technical B. Students who have graduated from the Community High Schools can be admitted to the craft courses at the Technical Institutes on an individual basis depending upon their performance.[7]

The post "academic secondary school" examination has been changed from the Ordinary and Advanced Levels of the General Certificate of Education Examinations, conducted by London University, to the Caribbean Examination Council (CXC). These new examinations may be taken only after a student has completed five years in a Multilateral School. These new examinations are of two types—The General Proficiency Certificate and the Basic Proficiency Certificate. The General Proficiency Examination can be graded on five levels: 1) Grade I—comprehensive knowledge of the syllabus, 2) Grade II—working knowledge of most aspects of the syllabus, 3) Grade III—working knowledge of some aspect of the syllabus, 4) Grade IV—limited knowledge of a few aspects of the syllabus, and 5) Grade V—insufficient evidence on which to base a judgment. If a student passes the examinations at a Grade I or Grade II level, his progress will be considered comparable to the Ordinary Level of the General Certificate of Education, London. This level of work will be considered as satisfying both University and Faculty requirements for entrance to the University of Guyana. The subjects that the student can be tested in are English (literature is emphasized), mathematics, foreign language, natural and social sciences.

The basic Proficiency Examination may be taken in subjects which the students do not wish to pursue for further study. Temporarily, it was also an option for students registered for the Ordinary Level of the General Certificate of Education, London, but who are aware that their chances of passing that examination were not good. The University of Guyana may consider the Basic Proficiency Certificate as an appropriate admission requirment on an individual basis and with certain specifications on that student's University program.[8]

There is one other means by which a student may enter the University of Guyana. Mature applicants (those in their 26th year or older) may petition the Faculty Admissions Committee for admission to a degree, certificate or diploma course. Decisions are made on an individual basis and will be considered, provided that the student has a "good general education and relevant technical experience."

The University of Guyana has two sets of admissions criteria—general criteria for admission to the university as a whole, and special criteria determined by the individual faculties. The general university admission requirements are: 1) five subjects passed at the Ordinary Level of the General Certificate of Education, London, or five Grade I or II level passes on the Caribbean Examinations Council's test; 2) all students are required to work for the National Service and/or National Development —additionally, students may be required to serve at any time. The faculties at the University of Guyana are: Arts, Natural Sciences, Social Sciences, Agriculture, Education, and Technology. Each faculty has a detailed list of requirements for admission. The university has non-degree diploma courses in Public Administration, Public Communication, Technology, and a Higher Technical Diploma in Mining Engineering. There is also a Post-Graduate Diploma in Education. This program is open to those who have completed their degree and who are presently working in the field of education.[9]

It is important to note the significance of the National Service requirement, in which young boys and girls are assigned to co-educational work camps in the interior, where they clear jungle, pave roads, etc. Culturally, East Indians, in addition to the "old upper class" Portugese and Chinese, find this highly objectionable and generally forbid not only their daughters in particular but also their sons to take part in these programs. This point of view prevents the child from securing the kind of education necessary for employment and social stability. From independence until about 1974 these families were able to send their children abroad to study. However, the government has made it illegal to take any major sum of money out of Guyana (between 1975 and 1979 the legal amount was approximately seven U.S. dollars, per person, per year, without special permission from a government official; later, the amount was raised to U.S. $75). Additionally, it is illegal and punishable by imprisonment for a Guyanese citizen to have any money in bank accounts or investments outside of Guyana. Guyanese are legally allowed to leave the country with jewelry consisting of wedding rings, a watch and a pair of earrings for women. Thus, by effectively prohibiting the outward flow of capital and by enforcing work requirements which are a cultural anathema to a large section of the country, the government has either forced these individuals to leave Guyana or to reject their culture and socialization totally and to become members of this "new social order."

As the government has attempted to change and revolutionize the society (for the most part, this has been a quiet revolution). It has taken certain deliberate steps in modifying the educational system. All education from primary school through university is completely free. Most, if not all, schools are co-educational and all have been removed from the control of religious denominations, although qualified religious persons are still allowed to teach. Teachers are assigned to schools by the government. Although parents have some choice in selecting a primary school, children can later be reassigned. Of greater consequence is the fact that many textbooks are being published in Guyana, especially those dealing with the social sciences. The government has also devised a new system of political education mandatory at all schools because it has been made part of the examinations for entering secondary school as well as part of the Caribbean Council Examination.

The major theme of the social studies course is national policy. Important aspects of policy which are to be studied are assigned, although it is expected that these will be broadened. The first theme is "Understanding the National Environment and How the Environment Serves the People." This deals with resources and the government's rationale for ownership and control of resources. The second theme is "Workers' Contributions," emphasizing the importance of individual work, cooperation, self reliance, and leadership. The third is "Elements of Guyanese History," dealing with the common experience under socialism and nation-building in addition to constitutional development and the role of the working class, the Guyana Labor movement, and the struggle for suffrage and independence. The fourth theme is "The Structure and Function of Government," which describes the operations and functions of government, the leaders, and their roles. The fifth aspect is "The Political Process and Philosophical Considerations." This area deals with the present development of socialist practices and case studies of various Guyanese institutions to examine their individual progress toward socialism.[10]

With this understanding of the historical background of education in Guyana, we turn our attention to the contributions made by some few individuals to educating the population about health and illness through the indirect means of scientific research achievement, medical care application, and dedicated professional performance.

A Medical Research Conference

In 1959, Dr. George Giglioli, one of the pioneers of health education in emerging Guyana, presented a fascinating account of the experiences of a health officer, the factors that shape a researcher, and the intersection of theoretical and applied interests in medical research:

> I deeply appreciate the privilege of addressing you here today, as I feel that nobody can understand quite as well as I do what this meeting of the Standing Committee for Medical Research means to those interested in medical and public health research in this country. I say this because during the 36 years I have worked in British Guiana I have been confronted with a number of problems requiring research, and I have always had to tackle such tasks in what might be described as "superb isolation." Nobody within the Colony appeared particularly interested in my subjects so that opportunity for intelligent and stimulating discussion did not exist. Exchanges with workers in other countries —during the earlier years at least—were difficult. Before airmail became available, it took at least three months to get an answer to a letter. Distinguished scientists occasionally turned up but such visits, however stimulating, were just fleeting incidents.
>
> In Georgetown we have not been overworked in preparing for or attending medical conferences! I did not get here in time to attend the last one, as it took place in 1921, the year before I came to British Guiana.
>
> It is enough to cast one's eye around this hall to realize how things are changing; we have here with us today two very distinguished representatives of the Medical Research Council, Sir George Pickering and Professor A. C. Fraser; Dr. Lewthwaite, Director of the Institute of Medical Research at Kuala Lumpur in Malaysia; we have some consultants from W.H.O., a strong contingent from the Medical School of the University College of the West Indies; Dr. Wilbur Downs, Director of the Regional Virus Laboratory in Trinidad; Dr. Horace Gillette—incidentally a Guianese—Medical Services of all the Caribbean territories and a number of other distinguished visitors from the islands and the U.S.A.
>
> It is of the greatest importance to note that this large and authoritative medical congress is not an isolated occurrence, as, for instance, the Medical Conference of 1921. This is the fourth birthday of the Standing Committee for Medical Research and we have just concluded the fourth Scientific Medical Conference held in these territories since 1956.

Medical research workers in this vast area have had for the past years an opportunity to meet each other; they have followed from year to year new developments and progress in each territory; they have been able to discuss their problems formally and informally among themselves and with the experienced visitors from the U.K. and the University College of the West Indies. All this means continuity in exchange of views, continuity and extension of research projects, pooling of means and brains, and above all, the creation of that environment and climate in which the ideal of medical research can be implanted and take root, and latent capabilities and talent activated and developed.

The general aim of the Standing Committee for Medical Research is to foster scientific medical studies throughout this large and nearly virgin area; specifically, it aims to bring West Indians in increasing numbers into this field, not only because these territories will eventually have to provide for themselves their own needs, even in research, but also because it is *the trained man on the spot* living in constant contact with the local clinical and public health problems who is in the best position to carry out good field work. He knows the environment and has that possibility of continuity of observation and study which the short-term visitor from abroad can obviously not achieve.

The Standing Committee does not limit its activity to the organization of periodical conferences; in its annual meetings it examines research programs submitted by workers in this area and if necessary it may allocate grants in aid of the projects it has approved.

The number of projects submitted so far, however, has not been as large as had been hoped considering the size of the Caribbean area and the immense scope for original medical research which it presents. Nearly half the funds which were actually available have not yet been spent; this has been the source of some disappointment. Speaking for myself I can't say that I am either surprised or disappointed by this apparent lack of interest, for at the present stage I feel that it could hardly have been otherwise. It would be a grave mistake to allow oneself to become discouraged.

In the West Indies and in this country, the general social environment, as it exists today, and even more so as it was in the more or less recent past, does not present the conditions which are at all likely to bring about, stimulate and develop that enquiring and also disinterested frame of mind which is a basic ingredient in the make-up of any real scientist or medical researcher.

Research means a lot of hard and unremitting *work over and beyond* the routine of any busy medical man, be he employed in a laboratory, a hospital, a mining camp, a plantation or in private practice. In addition, research is certainly not a financial proposition!

There can be no doubt that some persons come into this world with an innate instinct and urge towards enquiry and research; they are not satisfied to accept what others take for granted; they want to know why and how things happen. In most cases, however, this frame of mind is acquired, and develops through contact, and more or less intimate association with persons engaged in or cultivating intellectual and research pursuits. It is probably at home that the first and deepest impressions are received and developed; obviously a child who grows up in a home full of books, where good reading and study is a habit, is in a better position to develop an inquisitive mind than his equally intelligent playmate belonging to a household where literature is missing or limited to illustrated magazines, comics and detective stories.

The secondary school is also without doubt a fertile nursery of future scientists; an imaginative science of biology master who feels his subject may influence the sensitive mind of a youngster more deeply, effectively and permanently than a whole medical faculty at a later stage when the student has embarked on his university studies, and has already made up his mind as to his future career. Conversely, a master who presents biology as an arid series of systematic classifications may instill in the subject an abiding horror for anything connected with this subject.

In this part of the world, most of our students proceeding to universities originate from families in which business, commerce and practical farming have been the main interests, often for generations.

In the secondary schools they meet boys and girls with an identical background and outlook; thus the opportunity for the exchange and development of ideas, which is so characteristic and important an educational factor in student life in all fully advanced countries, is inevitably limited. This explains why up to recently only two alternatives appeared to be entertained by our prospective university graduates; law or medicine, both being conceived purely and simply as practical professions.

Things, however, have been changing over the last ten or so years and such subjects as engineering, biology, chemistry, forestry, veterinary medicine, etc., are being taken up. The circle of persons with a scientific education is getting wider and more varied and the environment for the early germinating of research mindedness should be improving. This, however, is a slow process which takes time to develop.

Some misconceptions exist which tend to deter from medical research men who have the preparation, the ability and unrivaled opportunities for doing very valuable work. Some underestimate their own capabilities and value of their studies and experiences. They cannot be prepared to produce or publish their findings; very valuable contributions may thus be lost, sometimes forever, as in these days conditions change rapidly and observations which are easy today may be difficult or even impossible in a few years time.

Others set their sights too high and expect early and important results with practical applications from their work; they are not interested in detail and in findings which appear to have only scientific or academic interest. The distinction between what is practical and what is academic is highly fallacious, as what is only interesting knowledge today may acquire practical importance tomorrow. DDT was first discovered by a German chemist in 1876; it did not appear at the time to be of any particular importance. It was discovered for the third time during the last war—when its revolutionary residual insecticidal properties were established. The academic discovery of 1876 helped win the last war and has revolutionized the fight against malaria and other insect-borne diseases and agricultural pest control throughout the world.

In connection with academic and applied research, I would like to tell you as short story which concerns my own work in this country.

In 1931, when I was Medical Officer of the Demerara Bauxite Company, at Mackenzie, the process of washing bauxite ore was first introduced for the purpose of freeing it from clay and other impurities. Water was pumped from the Demerara River to the washing plant, and hence it drained into the forest at the back of the mill, eventually finding its way back to the river. A few months later, there was a steep increase in the number of malaria cases; on investigation we found very large numbers of the dangerous Anophiline malaria carrier breeding in ponds and puddles formed by the clarified water issued from the washer plant. Further studies showed that the black water of the Demerara River was very acid and this rendered it unsuitable for the breeding of dangerous mosquitoes; this same water, after being churned in the washers with bauxite and clay, became nearly neutral and an excellent breeding medium. This was the first observation connecting the distribution and incidence of malaria and its carrier with the reaction of ground waters in this country. This malaria outbreak at Mackenzie was controlled by building a high dam around the tailing pond and circulating the pond's water back to the washing plant as soon as it was settled. Thus the amount of water was limited and it was kept in constant movement; mosquito breeding was eliminated. An identical, but much graver malarial exacerbation occurred at Mackenzie during the war, when through production pressure the old tailing pond became inadequate and reversion to the original washing technique was imposed.

Studies on the relation of ground water reaction to *Anopheles* breeding were continued systematically on the sugar estates up to the beginning of the war, but no means were discovered to apply the knowledge so gained to practical malaria control.

At H.M.P.S. on the Mazaruni River, I found conditions exceptionally favorable for the study of the relations of soil types and geological formation to the various types of waters, brownstained and colorless, more acid and less acid, as all such types occurred in close proximity to each other in this area.

Unfortunately, however favorable environmental conditions might be, laboratory facilities were sadly lacking for the carrying out of controlled experiments to check on field observations; for instance, none of the traditional laboratory glassware was available. This shortage was overcome by the use of a certain type of intimate chinaware which for reasons unknown was available in abundant supply at H.M.P.S. These containers produced an imposing and quite original display in my improvised laboratory. Percolators were also necessary to test the effect of various types of soils on the waters flowing through them; admirable efficient apparatus was rigged up making use of long lengths of bamboo from which the *septa* had been chiseled out. These investigations continued for two years, but even so, we could devise no practical methods by which ground waters could be artificially acidified so as to eliminate the breeding of malaria mosquitoes. You must remember that at that time practical malaria control was based exclusively on water control and antiluvial measures.

Then in 1945, DDT came to British Guiana and by 1948 malaria had been eradicated from the inhabited coastland. A new question then confronted us; British Guiana being a continental country and not an island, did we have to go on indefinitely spraying every house in the rural and suburban areas from Charity on the Pomeroon to Crabwood Creek on the Corentyne? Could we interrupt spraying, and, if so, in which areas, for how long, and at what risk?

Our apparent academic studies of the past 25 years supplied the answer to these questions: the acid waters of the peaty pegasse swamps lying aback of the inhabited cultivated coastlands and the white sand formations lying still further inland with their acid black waters, constitute an impassable barrier against possible re-invasion of *Anopheles darlingi* from the forests of the interior. We could suspend spraying operations all along the coast, only maintaining "road blocks" of DDT, and spray houses on the river estuaries and on the minor water courses which, with their alluvial banks, could provide reinvasion routes for the mosquito from the interior. This policy has been in successful operation for over 9 years with a saving of several hundreds of dollars each year.

I have told you this story because it shows that research should be carried out as an end to itself; and that in field research, much can be accomplished with little or even with make-shift apparatus. There is, however, no make-shift or substitute for scientific curiosity and pertinacity!

I have tried to outline objectively some of the causes—as I see them—of the rather slow response to the efforts of our Committee. I wish to repeat, however, that I do not think there is cause for disappointment; I have no doubts on local talent and ability, but it will take time, here as it has elsewhere, to form that inquisitive and interested frame of mind which is unconditionally essential for all forms of sound and honest scientific research.[11]

Summary

The Emancipation Act was passed in 1833. After this Act, religious groups were allowed to enter British Guiana to establish churches and schools. By 1847, there were 101 denominational schools. Since there were not enough trained teachers to cope with the proliferation of schools, it took some time to rectify this imbalance. By the Educational Ordinance of 1855, schools were owned or operated by Christian denominations and the government agreed to maintain school buildings and pay teachers' salaries. A compulsory education law was passed in 1876, but it was not very effective because many parents preferred to send their children to work, which would bring them some additional income.

School attendance for the Indian population was only one per cent in 1890 and 50 per cent by 1921. The pattern of education was worked out after the British mode. Primary education was organized by denominational groups or proprietary schools. All secondary schools except Queen's and Bishop's were denominational. After independence, the government shaped the educational policy in such a way as to achieve its national goals such as national integration and socialism.

Guyana has profited greatly from scientific research and medical care applications to eradicate the scourge of malaria. Dr. George Giglioli made a unique contribution to health education in Guyana in that process.

5

Hansen's Disease in Guyana

Dr. Patricia Rose of the Ministry of Health in Guyana is a physician who has contributed enormously to the education of the Guyanese population in health care. Her research has focused on the diagnosis, treatment, and prognosis of Hansen's disease. In 1978, Dr. Rose presented a series of articles in the Georgetown *Sunday Chronicle* for the purpose of educating the population about Hansen's disease, which plagued a segment of the nation for many years. Some of her ideas on Hansen's disease (leprosy) are found in the following remarks.

Early Treatment Ensures Complete Cure

Last Sunday I wrote about bacteria with special reference to the Mycobacterium that causes Hansen's disease and, you will remember, that this is a unicellular micro-organism known as an obligate human parasite because it can only survive inside the human body.

Today I want to begin to describe the changes that take place in the body when the Mycobacterium becomes established in a suitable host. But before doing so I must stress that although this organism is harmful because it is capable of causing illness, this illness is only likely to occur in a small proportion of any given community.

Most of us will not develop any sign of illness, however, after we encounter these bacteria. It is possible that they are not very virulent or aggressive in their attempts to colonize us but it is more likely that men generally are provided with adequate mechanisms for identifying these particular invaders as harmful and deal with them appropriately before they have an opportunity to become established.

The changes to be described, then, will occur only in a minority group. This small group succumbs to an illness that is determined in a type by the quality of the individual's response to infection. Just as there are those who are completely protected (represented by the bulk of the population and resulting in no infection or challenge) so there are those who are completely incapable of making any response. In between these two extremes of "no disease" and overwhelming infection there exists a wide spectrum of illness with symptoms varying according to the degree of resistance inherent in the particular individual under challenge.

Let us consider first of all those people whose resistance is just short of perfect and who are, therefore, not completely protected. Such people will demonstrate signs of illness of a "highly resistant" type on encountering these bacteria. The first thing they will notice is a "spot" on the skin or rather an area of skin that is gradually losing its color and becoming more pale.

Usually this spot is round or oval in shape with a regular, neat nargin clearly dividing it from normal skin. Sometimes this margin is raised and looks rather like a ring of mosquito bites and this raised margin together with the circular shape of the "spot" tends to suggest a diagnosis of "ringworm."

However, a ringworm generally "itches" whereas the early lesions of high resistant Hansen's disease do not itch. In addition, the skin in an early Hansen's lesion loses its sensation as well as its depth of color. This loss of feeling is the hallmark of Hansen's disease.

Special

I explained in an earlier article that these Mycobacteria have a special liking for and are usually found in and around the nerves. These are bundles of very highly specialized tissue that connect our brain (the headquarters of our nervous system) with all parts of the body.

The function of this nerve tissue is to transmit messages both to and from our brain. Messages to the brain carry vital information and messages from the brain lead to action that is often dependent on this information.

The skin is very abundantly supplied with nerve endings sensitive to pain, temperature, touch and pressures and any damage or break in the continuity of the nerve fibres leaving the skin will interfere with the accurate transmission of information from these nerve endings.

This is what occurs in high resistant Hansen's disease; but the damage is caused not by the bacilli which are rarely, if ever, found; rather by the very aggressive and efficient response of the body defense system which throws out millions of defending cells that engulf the invading bacteria and disrupt the structure of the nerve fibres by the sheer weight of their numbers.

The typical early lesion of high resistant disease then is a pale, circular spot with a well marked margin. This spot exhibits some alteration of sensation from the time it first appears, while gradually progressing from an early "prickly" or "tingly" feeling when touched to a complete loss of sensation.

The exact color of early lesions varies somewhat according to the color of the normal skin. Lesions on dark skin are a very attractive copper color whereas those on lighter or white skins are a deep pink. The texture of the spot remains normal at first but as it ages it becomes gradually drier until the surface is quite rough. This increasing dryness is accompanied by a loss of hair from the area.

These spots grow slowly and are not accompanied by any of the warning signs of illness such as malaise, fever, headaches, etc. In fact, it is likely that the greater proportion are self-healing ones. Complications of a disastrous nature may occur with lightning rapidity and early treatment is simple and produces a complete cure. Even established loss of sensation reverts to normal if treatment is commenced soon enough.

A single spot signifies a high degree of resistance to infection. When several spots are present it can be assumed that the patient is less resistant and when many exist the disease is obviously of a systemic nature and the bodily resistance is insufficient to cope with the situation alone.

Patients Never Likely to Transmit Infection

Before the advent of antibiotics, it was customary to isolate patients with Hansen's disease in a vain attempt to isolate the illness with them.

Nowadays it is considered more effective to isolate the bacteria instead by treating the patients with drugs. Most patients have a high level of resistance and require treatment only to protect themselves from the harmful effects of nerve damage. A great deal of the treatment in these cases is directed towards calming down the violence of the body's response to invasion and protecting the nerves at risk while administering antibiotics which enable the body to eliminate the bacteria in a less traumatic manner.

Patients with little or no resistance to infection need treatment both to heal themselves and to ensure that the infection does not spread to others. In these cases, a bactericidal drug (one that kills bacteria outright) is given during the first few weeks of treatment in addition to dapsone. This means that in a matter of hours or days the patient becomes quite incapable of passing on the infection to anyone else. Obviously, the earlier the treatment starts, the fewer bacteria there are to be disposed of and the shorter the time interval required to conquer the infection.

You will remember that only a small proportion of any given population is likely to succumb when attacked by this particular micro-organism. Most of us are quite capable of dealing with it should we encounter it. This relatively low level of population susceptibility, coupled with the bactericidal properties of the treatment available, should enable the level of infection within the community to be reduced to a minimum. The problem, as with most other chronic infections, remains a problem because it is not tackled vigorously and promptly when it first appears.

From every point of view, early treatment is desirable. It completely protects individuals from the consequences of nerve damage and at the same time reduces the level of infection within the community.

Congenital and hereditary conditions invariably arouse interest and speculation and I am always being asked whether Hansen's disease is congenital. It is not. There is a very wonderful organ filtering the blood that passes between the mother and her baby in the womb; it is called the placenta. By means of this organ the baby is supported and fed during its life before birth and one of the most important functions of the placenta is to prevent any harmful bacteria from reaching the baby. Very few micro-organisms manage to pierce this almost impregnable barrier and Mycobacteria are not among them.

Hereditary complaints are passed on within families by abnormalities in the genes. Hansen's disease is not transmitted in this way. It is thought likely that susceptibility to infection may be inherited, perhaps a faulty mechanism for identifying and reacting to certain pathogenic bacteria.

Hansen's disease then is a bacterial infection caused by a micro-organism that is so perfectly adapted to living within man that it is unable to exist elsewhere. It is neither a congenital nor hereditary disease and the majority of the population can respond to its challenge without ever becoming ill. The susceptible minority will only suffer nerve damage if treatment is delayed or neglected.

As with most disease, early treatment is simpler, shorter, and produces the best results. However, the insidious development of the illness and the absence of generalized symptoms such as fever and malaise tend to encourage patients to wait too long before seeking help.

It cannot be emphasized enough that there are adequate supplies of drugs in Guyana for treating every patient. Everyone can expect a complete cure but the chances of cure without residual disability will diminish the longer the treatment is postponed.

The nerves that transmit informational material to our brains and conduct directional messages from them are very easily damaged. In untreated Hansen's disease they may be compressed, blurring the slow but relentless progression of the illness, or suddenly destroyed in an acute phase.

As I explained [previously], these complications do not occur early in the course of the illness and can be completely avoided by early treatment. In the absence of early and adequate treatment, however, serious destruction of nerve tissue is inevitable in most cases and therefore, as I stressed in an earlier article, it is not wise to watch spots in hope that they may be self-healing.

Delay in treatment results in loss of sensation and it leads to extensive damage to the hands or feet or both, according to the nerves involved. Because these damaged limbs are frightening to some of us and because this damage is entirely preventable, I want to discuss it in some detail.

The initial injury is usually a burn or a scald but may be an infected finger following a thorn or splinter in the flesh. Because superficial feeling is lacking the wound is not usually noticed by the patient until it has become badly infected and an abscess has formed and even then the pain is not sufficient to ensure that the finger is kept at rest.

When feeling is present, rest is automatic because the finger hurts more when it moves. This rest is the most essential part of the healing process as it allows the decalcified finger bones to be completely recalcified and reshaped so that the finger retains its habitual contour.

The finger bones are decalcified by the flushing of blood which is necessary for the healing of the abscess; but, without rest, normal recalcification does not follow and although the abscess eventually heals the patient is left with a shorter finger. When this process is repeated several times the shortening of the finger becomes more and more obvious until, in extreme cases, the whole finger is lost. Such damage is completely avoided by early treatment. Care of the hands and especially immediate attention to all injuries however trivial, can completely prevent any loss of tissue.

Insensitive fingers are easily burnt during the performance of the normal household tasks, particularly dining, cooking and also by holding on for too long to cups of hot liquid such as tea or coffee or by smoking cigarettes too close to the filter. Fingers may be damaged by simple repetitive actions such as turning radio switches, handling sharp keys, opening tin cans and so on. In fact, without intact sensory nerves, man is isolated from his environment and simple, homey surroundings become hostile and ordinary, everyday tasks become hazardous.

The cycle of injury, infection, abscess and loss of tissue is secondary to the loss of sensation resulting from the interruption of the nerve pathway to the brain. it can be regarded as the end result of untreated or inadequately treated illness but the bacteria responsible for this trouble are not around at the site of the damage. They are, or were far away inside the superficial nerve trunk, supplying the affected limb. There is no need, therefore, to be afraid that any of these damaged limbs can spread the infection to others. Neglect of injury spells disaster, but only for the patient concerned, not for his neighbors.

We have become so accustomed to living in a society where antibiotics are freely available for the treatment of infection that we tend to forget what life was like without these wonderful drugs. Over the last 30 years they have been involved in a quiet revolution that has completely changed the face of medicine.

Prior to the 1970s recovery from infection depended on the resistance of the individual. Treatment consisted in keeping the patient at rest so as to conserve all his energies for fighting off the infection and bolstering his general health by various supportive measures.

If you were unfortunate enough to contract one of the serious infections of childhood such as scarlet fever, the outlook was grim indeed; a boil on the face could lead to septic meningitis with invariably a fatal outcome; childbirth fever caused many deaths as did typhoid fever and such infections affected people in every walk of life. Prince Albert, the Prince Consort and husband of Queen Victoria, died of typhoid fever when the science of enviromental health was in its infancy.

Surgical practice too has been affected by the revolution. Before the introduction of antibiotics, infections of the hand or fingers too often resulted in abscess formation.The abscess had to be opened when "ripe" and this operation was preceded and followed by days of poulticing and painful dressings.

Among the first of the wonder drugs were sulphonamides and dapsone, the drug used for the treatment of Hansen's disease, is closely related to them. It is usually administered by mouth in tablet form, is well absorbed and relatively small amounts are effective so that it is not necessary to take more than one tablet daily. However, in order to maintain steady blood levels it is necessary to take the daily tablet very regularly. Like the sulphonamides, dapsone is bacteriostatic—it prevents the bacteria from dividing and gives the body defenses a chance to get rid of the bacteria. You will remember that these particular micro-organisms have a long generation time and are very well adapted to life inside man. They are not easy to get rid of and to be effective, treatment MUST be taken not only regularly but also over a long period of time. This is obviously a disadvantage and people sometimes become disheartened at the thought of having to continue treatment for so long. However, the results of adequate treatment are so good that it is well worth persevering. One must remember, also, that the changes in the skin have taken a long time to develop and the healing process is likely to be equally slow.

Besides dapsone there are a few other drugs that are sometimes useful. They may be given in addition to dapsone and it is now considered advisable for low resistant patients to take two drugs at the same time. Whatever drugs are used the ingredients for success remain the same—regularity of treatment and perseverance. There are no short cuts.

Naturally, the earlier the treatment starts the smoother the course of the illness and the better results. Treatment started at a later stage will take a longer time and the normally tranquil healing process may be interrupted by episodes of acute illness.

The spot or spots on the skin in the high resistant form of Hansen's disease tend to be disregarded by the patient because there is no pain or irritation and the loss of sensation develops so slowly that it is not obvious unless the spot is at a site subject to trauma.

With the onset of an acute phase, however, the spot changes color, becoming progressively redder until it is a bright, blood red and at the same time it swells so that it stands out more obviously from the surface of the skin. These alarming changes occur very rapidly, in a few hours or days, the sudden swelling making the spot irritating and sometimes painful. Fortunately, such abrupt changes usually compel the patient to seek medical aid because if left untreated these spots will damage any nerve running through them. Nerves are very easily compressed by fluid in the tissues and if this acute swelling is not rapidly relieved there will be permanent loss of sensation in the skin of the area and if the spot lies nerar a nerve trunk its compression will lead to paralysis of the muscles served by that nerve. However, even after the onset of paralysis, correct treatment can still effect a cure if it is begun within days or preferably within hours.

Patients with low resistant disease are subject to similar acute phases and also to rheumatic type of illness with fever and pains in the hands and feet sometimes accompanied by irritation, reddish bumps that appear on the skin overnight and fade during the daytime. These bumps resemble large mosquito bites, last a few days only and occur in successive crops. They may be accompanied by pain in the eyes which is always a serious moment as it heralds the onset of iritis which will lead to blindness if untreated.

In all forms of the disease episodes of acute illness are periods of great danger. They do not occur early and indicate that the patient has been ill for some years. Adequate treatment can still effect a cure but delay in treatment at this stage will lead to permanent disability.

In any community there will be a few people who are likely to be susceptible to the more generalized form of Hansen's disease.

The exact reason for the lack of resistance against this particular infection is not known but it has been suggested that these people are constitutionally unable to identify these micro-organisms as invaders.

The bacteria are, thus, able to multiply freely within the tissues without being attacked by the body's defense system.

This bacterium thrives best at fairly cool temperatures and is generally found in the cooler areas of the body—in the deeper layers of the skin, inside the nose and in the front section of the eye.

Early changes are most easily seen in the skin which develops a number of symmetrically distributed spots. Unlike those of the high resistant disease there are many spots and they do not have a distinct margin. These spots are never raised. This makes them much more difficult to see.

When the spots first appear they are plentiful on the trunk as well as on the limbs. They often appear like large raindrops but as they grow they merge into one another to make layers or "sheets" of a coppery color. These can easily be confused with "lata" which is a very superficial "ringworm" that when rubbed becomes much more obvious and stands out clearly from the surrounding skin, displaying its superficial nature (unless it has been previously oiled). Rubbing a spot of lower resistant Hansen's disease, however, does not produce any change.

Invasion of the nose is proceeding at the same time as the growth of the bacteria in the deeper layers of the skin. In the nose the bacteria develop within the nasal mucous membrane, leading to an increase in secretions and some blockage of the nose. This does not disturb the patient at first as it is generally assumed to be due to "head cold" or sinusitis.

As you would expect, the spots of low resistance disease do not show any loss of sensation in the early stages. In the article on high resistant disease I explained that early loss of sensation is due to disruption of nerve fibres by the mass of defense cells that pour into the nerve to destroy the bacteria trying to establish themselves therein.

As the body in low resistance disease is unable to recognize the bacteria as a possible enemy, these defense cells are slow to accumulate (and when they do they are singularly unsuccessful in getting rid of the bacteria). Thus, there is no early nerve damage and consequently, no early loss of sensation.

In between the two extreme types of almost complete resistance and no resistance at all, lies a wide spectrum of illness with symptoms dependent of the severity of the interaction taking place between the bacteria and their host. In nearly every case, however, it is a change in the skin that first alerts the patient to the fact that something is wrong, although as I have explained earlier, the battle is actually being fought inside the nerves.

Regardless of the type of resistance mounted by the patients, the illness takes a long time to develop. It has been estimated that the latent or incubation period between infection and the first sign of disease may vary between two and seven or even more years. Both the long generation time and the generally high degree of resistance tend to prevent the early onset of the illness.

The highly resistant form of Hansen's disease is not accompanied by any sign of generalized infection—such as malaise, fever, headaches, etc. This is in keeping with the picture of almost complete control. The host, that is the body, is confining the invaders to one very small area and doing it so successfully that neighboring parts of the body and other body systems are not drawn into the battle. However, the lower the resistance becomes the more evidence there is of spread to other parts of the body and patients with little or no resistance will eventually begin to experience more general signs of illness such as fever, fatigue, etc.

In the last two articles I have been describing the early signs of the disease. Next I want to talk about the likely outcome in cases that remain untreated but, before doing so, I will give a brief description of the type of treatment available.

It is very important always to keep in mind the following points:

First, we are talking about a curable bacterial infection for which ample treatment is available, and second—like most infections, early treatment produces the best results.[1]

We shall now turn our attention to the role of physicians in Guyana —their social backgrounds, decisions to enter the field of medicine, and their attitudes toward the medical profession.

6

Physicians in Guyana

In this chapter we shall present information on the social backgrounds and some selected attitudes of physicians in Guyana. We shall further specify the contributions of Dr. George Giglioli, who did so much to improve the health of the Guyanese people.

In the middle 1960s and early 1970s, data were gathered in Guyana through questionnaires and attitude inventories. The purpose was to get some indication of how physicians who practice medicine in a newly emerging nation respond to some selected aspects of professional medical training.

The questionnaires and attitude inventories were given to a group of 45 physicians practicing medicine in Guyana. Additional data were obtained from extensive participant observation of members of the study group within their hospital settings, living quarters in the hospital compounds, dispensaries located in the various estates, and in informal social gatherings.

Characteristics of the Social Background of Guyanese Physicians

Social class position is an extremely subtle dimension of status, difficult to identify in a developing nation such as Guyana. Prior to independence, class distinctions were based primarily upon race and family positions of power or control in government and business enterprises. However, with the advent of independence, it seems as if greater emphasis has been placed upon profession or occupation, length and type of education, and amount of income as indices of class position. Given the shifting bases of social prestige, no attempt was made to rank the respondents according to social class position in the group, which is racially and ethnically heterogeneous in composition.

In general, however, the physicians in the study group mirror the position long held by practicioners of medicine in Guyanese society—a well-paid, high-status professional occupation. Sixty-six percent of the respondents are native born citizens of Guyana; almost 90 per cent of their mothers and fathers are also native born. The others in the sample are citizens either of the United Kingdom or of India.

The majority of the physicians are under 40 years of age, indicating that they followed a regular sequence of college and direct entry to medical school. About 20 per cent formed a cluster in having more years of practice in medicine as compared to others in the sample.

Although coming from relatively comfortable families, two-thirds of the physicians stated that they had economic problems while attending medical school. The data revealed that, although parents were the most important source of funds for attending medical schools, over two-thirds of the members in the study group depended on scholarships and fellowships to complete a substantial portion of their medical education.

Factors in the Decision on a Field of Practice

The decision of the physicians in the group to enter into a field of practice upon completion of their medical education was determined by the extent to which various factors had influenced their choice of practice as a career. In this study group, the most important source of influence affecting such a decision was said to be the physician's own intellectual interests. Once the decision had been made, parents, spouse, and clinical chiefs during internship encouraged the respondents to continue their hospital training beyond their internship. It is of interest to note that 65 per cent of the members in the study group made a final decision during their internship on how much hospital training they would obtain for the future of their career.

Physicians' Attitude Toward the Medical Profession

Medicine as a profession has some general features which are important in identifying a "good" medical student over and above one's knowledge of medicine and one's ability to apply such knowledge. There undoubtedly are other vital features, but the authors have limited their attention in this report to the following list:

(1) Ability to establish rapport with patients;
(2) Ability to discern and deal with social and psychological problems of patients;
(3) Ability to get along with the patient's family;
(4) Ability to get along with other medical students;
(5) Academic abilities as evidenced in examinations, recitations, written assignments, etc.

Together, these five features of medicine provide a basis for analyzing some attitudes of practicing physicians toward students who have chosen the medical profession as a career, the assumption being that the respondents are at the same time revealing their own judgment toward medicine. Within this framework, the ability to establish rapport with patients was ranked as most important by nearly 90 per cent of the members of the study group. The ability to get along with the family of the patient was ranked least important by the respondents.

Although the majority of the physicians asserted that the ability to establish rapport with patients was the most important feature in identifying a good medical student, they were also aware of some dangers in such relations to their professional role. About two-thirds agreed that "if you don't watch out, when you are in practice, patients will take advantage of you." The majority agreed that "one of the problems in getting friendly with patients is that they don't know where to 'draw the line,' and that patients often lose respect for you."

The respondents were also questioned regarding their feelings about the race, education, and religion of their patients in order to assess whether any of these factors could be influential in affecting a physician's judgment of a patient as a person. It is of interest to note that the respondents considered education as the most important factor, while the majority were emphatic in not considering race as important.

Another aspect of the physicians' attitude toward their profession, which may have a bearing on the future practice of medicine in the Caribbean area, is the degree of their satisfaction with medicine as a career. The factors which seemed to be most important in bringing about satisfaction are a) the opportunity to help patients and b) the opportunity to utilize skilled techniques. The factors which seemed to be least important in bringing about greater satisfaction are a) financial reward and b) status in the community.

We have seen, therefore, that physicians in the group indicated that the most vital feature in identifying a good student- physician, over and above the knowledge of medicine and ability to apply such knowledge, is the ability to establish rapport with patients. It would appear that a statement of Professor Michael Beaubrun on the need for physicians to *understand* their patients is germane to this finding in this study. Professor Beaubrun asserted that

> in a culture in transition from religio-magic thinking to scientific, pragmatic thinking, it is most important that not only the psychiatrist but every doctor be taught the social anthropological background of the patients with whom he deals and how these patients perceive him; for a

doctor from the middle class or social elite is usually surprisingly unaware of his patients' beliefs and value system.[1]

Hence, it would seem that greater emphasis should be given to the importance of psychology, sociology, and cultural anthropology during the preclinical years of study in medical school.[2]

Outstanding Physicians in Guyana

Having briefly presented the background and selected attitudes of almost 50 physicians in Guyana, it is now appropriate to highlight the important contributions of three of the most outstanding physicians in the country from a historical perspective. The first of these is Dr. George Giglioli.

Dr. George Giglioli

We have previously noted that Dr. George Giglioli was one of the most outstanding physician-researchers in Guyana. In June 1966, he gave a very vivid account of his pioneering work on health and illness in Mackenzie—the center of the bauxite industry in Guyana. Dr. Giglioli noted in his talk, "Retrospect: Mackenzie 1922–1932":

> If at any stage in our life we attempt to look forward for forty or fifty years, it feels as if we were trying to look into eternity; in retrospect, however, time presents a completely different dimension and memories of people and events of half a century or more ago are often as vivid as if they had occurred yesterday. Obviously, a great deal is irreparably lost and forgotten. Of this, however, we are unconscious. In contrast, what survives in our memories appears clear and fresh, and I should like to say nearly as tangible as a good collection of brilliant color transparencies.
>
> In November 1922, when my wife and I, as a newly married couple, arrived at Mackenzie, the plant had been closed for approximately three years, after operating on a very small scale, for a few months during the First World War. Deterioration had set in on a large scale and second growth bush had taken over much of the original clearing. The main dock on which we landed had to be negotiated with care and we were told that only a few days previously, the new Chief Accountant had stepped off the steamer only to land on a rotten board and into the Demerara River. Rehabilitation work, however, was in full swing and over 1,000 men were then employed at Mackenzie.

The plant proper comprised the power house, the crusher, drying and storage buildings with their tall conveyors, the M.U. store, the General Office, the old hospital and a very dilapidated machine shop.

Cockatara village was quite small, extending between the Cockatara Creek and the site where the recreation hall was later erected. There were only four or five family cottages of fair standard, and some barracks used as 4-family quarters. Most of the buildings were bunk houses with only two or three bachelor quarters. Most of the men who worked at the mine lived in the bunk houses at Three Friends. A large proportion of the labor force (was made up of) West Indians from St. Lucia, Dominica and Grenada. They were very steady and hard workers. Few, however, had their families with them so that at that time Mackenzie women and children were scarce.

To reach Watooka Staff Quarters from the Office and Plant, one followed a rough unpaved track through thick second growth bush close to the railway; the Watooka creed was crossed on a very rickety bridge. During the rains, which were very heavy and continuous at the time of our arrival, this track became a quagmire. Wheel traffic at Mackenzie in 1922 consisted of a single donkey cart which delivered ice and supplies from the Company's Ration Store at Cockatara. The staff village itself consisted of some twelve cottages disposed symmetrically on each side of the single road and the club house where some bachelors were housed. Beyond the club, there was thick second growth bush. The main clearing extended from the river to railway; beyond that, there was high forest.

The staff houses were built on exactly the same pattern. They were closely spaced and all were painted a dull, dark gray. Each house consisted of two bedrooms, a sitting room-gallery, a bathroom, a pantry and a kitchen. They had been erected as temporary quarters for the early prospectors and construction personnel. Close to the creek, Watooka House was being built as the manager's residence on pillars which had originally been intended for a very ambitious two-story hospital which, however, never materialized.

At the time of our arrival, the staff consisted of 12 men, there were only 6 ladies in the camp and 3 children. The manager was Blaicksley Barnes, an exceptionally fine American engineer who was very much liked by all who worked under him as he was competent, humane and fair; and this earned him the nickname "Down the River" Barnes, for the many he dispatched back to Georgetown for repatriation. One character who arrived intoxicated was not even allowed to get off the river steamer. He returned to England by the same ship which had brought him out. Much to our regret, Barnes was transferred to Surinam in 1925. During the remaining seven years we spent at Mackenzie things were never what they had been during his regime.

Tennis and swimming in the river off the old club Stelling were the main recreation. My wife swam twice a day throughout the ten years we were at Mackenzie, and our boys took to the water as soon as they were one year old, and eventually developed into excellent swimmers. The youngest swam across the river and back at the age of 4. I followed in a corial and had him at the end of a long fishing line . . . just in case. Sundays we usually passed hunting and trapping in forest and canoeing in the creeks.

The hospital I found on arrival was a rough wooden structure consisting of a twelve-bed ward for male patients only, a dispensary, a treatment room and a tiny office. Its staff comprised a dispenser, a male nurse, a helper and a cook. Equipment was rudimentary and there were no proper facilities for sterilization. In contrast, I was rather startled to find a set of instruments for advanced bone and skull surgery! The construction of the plant and railway was completed in the course of 1923. Early in the following year, we had a visit of inspection by Mr. Arthus Davis, President and Founder of Alcoa, which was at that time Demba's parent company. This visit marked the turning point in the history of Mackenzie, as it resulted in a firm decision to continue and expand mining operation. It then came to light that work during the previous 18 months had been essentially tentative and exploratory to decide whether Mackenzie should or should not be closed down for good. As Mr. Barnes told us at a dinner, little had we realized how precarious our jobs had been up to that day.

I had a short interview with the omnipotent Mr. Davis and emerged with instructions to prepare plans for the building and equipping of a new hospital. On an estimate of $80,000 and with instructions to plant semen trees all along the new road connecting Watooka with the plant, Mackenzie then might have an avenue comparable to Georgetown's Main Street. The avenue was planted a few weeks later with several dozens of semen seedlings sent up from the Botanical Gardens. Some of these trees are now quite large, but growth had been uneven and replacements have not been made. I doubt that the avenue as it exists today would come up to Mr. Davis' high expectations.

With the prospect of expanding operations, it was suggested that an assistant medical officer should be appointed. This seemed a good idea considering the difficulties experienced in sending surgical and seriously injured patients to Georgetown, and also the very poor standard of surgery then available in the country. I advised that a specialized surgeon should be brought out, as this would fill a much more urgent and specific need. I thus got in touch with an old boyhood and university friend and in November 1924, Dr. Romiti arrived in Mackenzie to operate on his first case—a partial amputation of a crushed foot—within an hour of his stepping off the river steamer.

The new hospital was inaugurated in May 1925. Its first function was to accommodate most of the V.I.P.s who attended the official opening. The machine shop struck a commemorative aluminum medal for the occasion.

The hospital comprised male and female wards, private rooms, and an out-patient section, and was well equipped for the treatment of medical, surgical, and maternity cases. It was adequately staffed for this purpose, and had a good x-ray as well as an excellent laboratory.

In 1926, I selected a boy, then an assistant teacher in the Christianbury Scots Church School, to train as a laboratory technician. This was Mr. Samuel Ramjattan who has been my constant and valued associate over the past forty years at Mackenzie, on the sugar estates in the Malaria Research Unit, throughout the Malaria Eradication Campaign. Others I wish to remember for their fine work are: Mr. Norman Stanton, the late Mr. James Jack, the late Mr. Caesar Nelson, Mr. Dickie, Matron Enid Chow, Nurse Pearcy and the late Mrs. Fred Proctor, at that time Nurse Crawford.

Medical and public health problems at Mackenzie were varied. Malaria prevailed and we all paid tribute to it repeatedly. As everywhere in this country it constituted the background on which every other disease seemed to evolve.

Malaria is most frequently aggravated by human activities. We evidenced this at Mackenzie in 1923, when the practice of washing the bauxite ore to free it from clay impurities was introduced for the first time. Millions of gallons of water were pumped from the Demerara River through the washers. This water then drained off into the forest at the back of the mill and eventually found its way back to the river through the Watooka and Cockatara creeks. The incidence of malaria in Cockatara and Watooka rose very steeply. We found that churning the river water with bauxite and clay, rendered it much less acid and thus made it a much more favorable medium for mosquito production. To meet the situation, a large area at the back of the mill was utilized to serve as a tailing pond. The same water, after sedimentation, was pumped back through the washers again, and again was kept in constant circulation which proved effective.

During the war, with greatly increased output, the tailing pond proved inadequate and the reversion to the old continuous one-way pumping became necessary. A large area of forest at the back of Mackenzie was deeply flooded. This resulted in a grave increase in malaria morbidity, which proved intractable till the advent of DDT in 1946. Hydraulic mining, also practiced at Mackenzie, had an identical effect in mosquito and malaria incidence. In 1925, a very severe malaria epidemic swept the whole district. Conditions along the river were so serious that a launch dispensary service was established, visiting settlements on alternate days from many miles above and below Mackenzie. With Dr. Ozzard and the late Dr. Moonsammy, I traveled as far as the Great Falls visiting every house and settlement. In an Akawayo Indian village at Nabura, everyone was ill and it was difficult to bury the dead who still lay in their hammocks. Dr. Ozzard contracted malaria on this trip which contributed to his death shortly after his return to Georgetown. During this outbreak, black water fever became quite frequent and some one hundred cases were treated at Mackenzie hospital. Bright's disease or chronic nephritis was also very common at Mackenzie, as elsewhere in the country, affecting children and young people. We discovered that this so-called "endemic nephritis" in British Guiana was caused by long untreated infection with the Querton parasite. This meant that this very fatal condition was both curable and preventable. It has in fact disappeared with the eradication of malaria.

Hookworm affected over 60 per cent of Mackenzie residents and was even more frequent and severe in the river population. It was controlled in 1924 by treating everybody in the course of two days. Workers were treated on the job, and families in their homes. We used what was then a new drug, carbon tetrachloride. It was very effective but has since been superseded by safer preparations. This campaign evolved without a hitch. I can remember only one very minor incident in the Electrical Workshop where both the electrician foreman and his assistant refused to take the medicine. There was an argument and I cannot recall if the drug was finally swallowed or not. Perhaps the chairman of the electricity corporation could refresh my memory. The results of this early campaign were maintained by sanitation and by treating systematically all newcomers to Mackenzie.

In 1932, the great economic world depression hit Mackenzie; curtailing operations and finally suspending them. Most of the staff was laid off, myself included. During the past ten years great strides had been made in the reorganization of the industry and in public health conditions. The foundations were being laid for the great expansion which became necessary during the war years.

We left Mackenzie in June 1932.[3]

Dr. Carlyle Miller

Dr. Carlyle Miller was a pastor of the Baptist Church in Guyana. He studied medicine and practiced his profession for several years in the United States. During his stay in America he obtained a grant from the Executive Board of his church to build a hospital in Guyana. He established the hospital at Long Creek, which is just half way between Georgetown and Linden. Apart from general health care, the hospital looks after maternity cases and provides pre- and post-natal care. Dr. Miller was ably assisted by Erma, his wife, and Dorothy Bavghems, a nurse. He felt that the hospital would flourish for many years to come.[4]

Dr. Enid Denbow

Dr. Enid Denbow was born in Guyana. After completing her secondary education, she joined the staff of the Georgetown Hospital as a nurse-probationer. Having successfully completed her nursing education, she applied for a job as a laboratory technician and was rejected. She later entered Harvard University as a pre-medical student. In 1955, she was graduated in medicine from Women's Medical College of Pennsylvania, and in 1956 she returned to Guyana and joined the Georgetown Hospital staff. From there, she went to Britain to specialize in internal medicine, cardiology and neurology. In July 1973, she was awarded a fellowship to Johns Hopkins University in Baltimore. In 1977, Edinburgh University conferred on her the F.R.C.P. (Fellow of the Royal College of Physicians) for her contributions to medicine in the Commonwealth Caribbean. Dr. Denbow is considered one of the hardest working physicians in Guyana. Apart from practicing medicine she holds many other responsible jobs.[5]

Dr. Raymond L. Warpeha

An American physician, Dr. Raymond L. Warpeha, has contributed enormously to the health care institution in Guyana. He is the director of Loyola University of Chicago Medical Center's Burn Center, and specializes in plastic and reconstructive surgery.

Dr. Warpeha has performed several operations at the Mercy Hospital in Georgetown. On one of his visits, Dr. Warpeha noted that "one boy, a two year old, had a cleft-palate and another, an eight-year old, had marked deformities of his hands as a result of burns he sustained as a very small child."

According to Dr. Warpeha, "the youngster with the deformed hands had no use of the right hand, and very little use of the left hand because of severe scar tissue. Both operations were successful." In addition, while there, he also saw a number of other patients on a consulting basis, and lectured on surgical management of the cleft palate.

Dr. Warpeha was the first American physician in his specialty to treat patients in Guyana. He noted that "plans would be made to invite one of the surgeons in Georgetown to come to Loyola University Medical Center to be trained in plastic and reconstructive surgery."

Patients and Physicians

Physicians, during the colonial years, enjoyed high status and prestige among the general population. In the villages, the physician was looked upon as one of the most respected persons in the community. He lived in one of the most expensive homes, with a large number of servants, a chauffeur, and a gardener, all provided for by the colonial government. His surgery facilities would be located on the first floor of his mansion and each day his office would be filled with patients who had traveled from far off villages and estates to receive medical help. Men, women, and children would sometimes walk barefoot for miles to obtain their bottle of medicine or box of pills from the doctor. In many instances, the doctor would have a dispenser (pharmacist assistant) working for him in his office. If the physician were elderly, then the dispenser would be trained by the doctor himself. The dispenser's job was to prepare the tablets and/or liquid medicine for the patients who had already seen the doctor perhaps three hours earlier. The wait in the physician's office in a village was indeed a test of patience for the afflicted person. In some instances, patients would leave in disgust and take their chances of recovery or death.

Repeatedly, a story was told that patients who did not follow the instructions of a particular physician were treated in a rather unusual manner. To make a patient respond to the doctor's order, a dose of castor oil was given in the surgery. The patient was told to rest for several minutes after the castor oil was taken. As soon as the castor oil was about to become active in the body, the patient was told to return home—usually by walking. Before the patient reached home, it was time for a bowel movement! After such an experience, the patient took great care in following the doctor's instruction.

In Guyanese culture the hospital is viewed as a very threatening place. It is a place to die rather than to be healed. Thus, if a physician, especially in the villages, informs a patient that surgery is necessary and that it has to be performed in the hospital, this information is viewed with tremendous fear and anxiety. The patient and members of the immediate family are perturbed day and night. Members of the family can become emotionally ill, the trauma lasting until the patient returns home in a healthy condition. If the patient dies, in some instances blame is attributed to the physician who had sent their loved one to a hospital "in town." If such is the case, the physician is viewed as incompetent and he is sometimes called "poor hopes"—meaning that if a patient goes to him for help, there is very little hope for recovery. Sometimes, the nickname "poor hopes" is given to a physician during his entire practice. If the physician moves to another village, friends and family of a deceased patient would communicate that information to the people of the village and the physician's name would remain the same—"poor hopes."

The physician who practiced as a government medical officer in a village also had to visit several outlying districts on various occasions. If the doctor was expected on a certain day, the patient's family would place a red flag in front of the house to indicate that someone was ill and that the physician should stop and visit the patient. Friends, neighbors, and other family members would congregate to meet the doctor, help him with his black bag, and direct him to the sick person. A doctor's presence in a patient's home created an atmosphere of awe and concern. If the physician was respected by the community, the family would be optimistic concerning the sick person's recovery. The doctor would be showered with repeated "thank yous" from the moment the patient was diagnosed and treated until the black bag was safely placed on the back seat of the automobile.

Summary

We have attempted to study the social backgrounds and some selected attitudes of physicians in Guyana. Before independence, class distinction was based on race or color, but now it is increasingly based on education, occupation and income. Two-thirds of the physicians had economic problems while attending medical school, and most of them depended on scholarships and fellowships to complete their studies.

78 Society and Health in Guyana

Once a medical student has finished his studies, his success is seen as depending on his attitude toward his patients. The ability to establish rapport with patients is ranked as important by nearly 90 per cent of the physicians interviewed. Most reject any discrimination.

Dr. Giglioli's contribution to Guyana's health services ranks high in the annals of Guyana history. In one of his talks about Mackenzie, he noted the hardship he and his wife endured. When he landed there he found a rough wooden structure called a hospital with twelve beds. Equipment was rudimentary. A new hospital was opened in May 1925 to fight malaria. As the great depression of 1932 hit Mackenzie, Dr. Giglioli was forced to leave in June 1932. Dr. Carlyle Miller and Dr. Enid Denbow have provided outstanding medical service to Guyana. Dr. Raymond L. Warpeha was the first American physician and surgeon in his specialty (plastic and reconstructive surgery) to treat patients in Guyana. Patient responses to medical care have been influenced by earlier years of hospitals and negative experiences of relatives or friends.

7
Folk Medicine Practices in Guyana

Guyana, like many developing nations in the Caribbean area, is steeped in the traditional use of folk medicine for healing. Because of the influence of East Indian and African cultures, many rural residents continue to use local remedies which have had their roots in the "old country." Although folk medicine and its remedies have been on the decline for years, their impact resonates even today.

Among some East Indian people, for example, vomiting and pain in the abdomen are often believed to be due to *Nara*. The family of the patient calls in a local healing expert, man or woman, depending upon the sex of the patient. The sick person is told to lie flat on the floor, and coconut oil is briskly rubbed from the head to the feet. The joints of the knees, arms and neck are cracked and the abdomen above the navel is tied with string several times before the patient is considered to be cured. The local healer, in order to make sure that the patient is well, takes a piece of string and measures the abdomen from the chest to the navel.

The common folk remedy for headache is to grind small onions into a paste, which is applied directly to the forehead. Toothaches are usually treated by placing either tobacco or eucalyptus oil on the suspected tooth. Oil is an important ingredient in remedies for various aches. If ants or other insects enter the ear, warm salt water or warm oil is poured into the ear to kill the insect and dislodge it.

Swellings due to sprains are also treated at home with ground medicinal herbs. Dislocated joints are massaged and set by certain persons who are believed to possess a special skill for such injuries. Minor cuts are also treated with ground oinions. Salt, used as a disinfectant, is also rubbed on cats and other small animals.

For coughs, a homemade preparation is made of sliced onions mixed with sugar. Colds and simple fevers are treated with a preparation made of dried ginger. Laxatives, such as epsom salts, are taken to "clean the system" in order to avoid fevers. In the case of constipation, tobacco or soap are used as suppositories.

Folk medications are used for childhood diseases like chicken pox, measles, and mumps, the most common in this country. For chicken pox, neem leaves are ground into a paste and applied to the eruptions on the skin, and the sick person is also given a bath in water mixed with the liquid extract of the neem leaves. Measles are usually allowed to run their course, but a special variety of plantains is sometimes eaten to bring out the rashes completely, allowing them to disappear at a faster rate.

Snake bites are rather common in rural areas, and it is commonly believed that if a person is bitten by a snake the punctured skin area should be sucked in order to draw the venom from the bloodstream of the stricken person.

Mental illness is often associated with the supernatural, hence a religious factor plays an important role in its cure. This belief is present among Hindus and Christians. Hindus have special prayer services, such as *poojas* and *mantras*, in which the patient is made to do various things such as crawl and rub pictures depicted on the floor. At the end of the curative ceremony, the patient falls unconscious and it is believed that the evil spirit will quickly leave the body. Another treatment for mental illness is the continuous pouring of cold water on the head of the patient — perhaps in the belief that it brings calm to the troubled mind.

In addition to these treatments for specific illnesses, there are also folk prescriptions for beauty treatments. For example, after delivery of a baby, an East Indian mother is made to consume a preparation of rice mixed with tumeric powder and coconut oil to give her good color. Tumeric powder is also rubbed over the body before taking a bath in order to acquire a certain color for the skin.

Similarly, the newborn child is given a preparation made of a little gold dust mixed in breast milk which is supposed to give a "good complexion" and a sweet voice to the child, especially if the child is a girl. A newborn baby is also rubbed each day with coconut oil warmed over the fireside. While the mother sits on the floor, with feet stretched out, the baby is placed on her feet and vigorously rubbed with them. The child is seen to enjoy such activity, especially with the mother singing to the child during the massaging. This procedure is supposed to straighten out the skull and facial bones of the newborn so that the child can grow and develop into a beautiful human being.

In many parts of the country, people utilize the services of the "bush doctor," who prescribes his remedies with apparent success. Orell, for example, is a riverside community of some 800 healthy and prolific persons. A trained nurse-midwife ministers to the needs of pregnant women. Aside from the pregnant women, everyone else goes to the bush doctor.[1]

It has been reported that "bush yaws" is an infectious "skin cancer" caused by a fly found in some areas of the Guyana hinterland. This fly resembles an ordinary housefly, but its bite transmits a virus which gets into the bloodstream. It has so baffled medical doctors that no one has ever cured it successfully. Corporal Clement Holder of the Guyana

Folk Medicine Practices in Guyana 81

Defense Force has reportedly cured three men suffering from "bush yaws" by using local herbs. These three patients seemed to have used all kinds of ointments, but in vain. Holder claims that he learned this herbal cure from Dr. Grewal and Dr. DeMel. The Guyanese acclaim Clement Holder as the "bush doctor miracle man."[2]

Charles Kyte, a Guyanese physician affiliated with the Tree of Life Institute in New York City, has recommended local herbs such as "bird pepper" celery seeds for the treatment of arthritis and rheumatism. He has claimed that anemia can be cured by using molasses and poor circulation by bird pepper and parsley root. A list of folk herb remedies prepared by Dr. Kyte appeared in the *Sunday Chronicle* (Guyana newspaper) on November 19, 1978.[3]

Tulchand Singh, a 27 year-old Guyanese, claims to have cured five people not through medicine but "through prayers and understanding of the spiritual centres." He is said to have given sight to Pooran Singh, a 23 year-old farmer. Sursattie, a 31 year-old deaf woman, says she is able to hear after this master's treatment. Hutiles was cured of his hernia. "Master" has restored sight to 70 year-old Henrietta Smight. "Master" has also set the bones of Cameron after a car accident. Tulchand Singh renders these services free of charge. Singh's reported cures have come to the attention of the medical doctors.[4]

Eileen Cox, a prolific writer for the *Sunday Chronicle*, encourages her largely urban readers to try home cures. She notes that Juliette De Bairachi Levy recommends anise seed as a powerful tonic. One teaspoon of the seed before meals three times daily is said to help digestion, improve appetite, alleviate cramps and nausea, and relieve flatulence and colic. Anise seed will also help to bring on menstruation and nursing mothers to produce more milk. A few seeds in a glass of hot milk will solve the problem of insomnia. Goldenseal is a described as a good tooth tonic. This herb is better than others to treat skin disease such as eczema and ringworm; moreover, it cures infections of the genital organs if taken orally. Garlic is used as an antiseptic, general tonic, worm deterrent, as well as for fevers and disorders of the blood, lungs, and tuberculosis. Garlic, raw in the form of a handful of leaves or taken dry, powdered or made into pills, reportedly protects one from whooping cough, asthma, high blood pressure, rheumatism, arthritis, and sciatica in addition to curing threadworms. Ginger, a good tonic for nerves and digestive organs, also relieves childbirth pains.[5]

Some physicians attached to the Public Hospital in Georgetown have at times condemned parents for going to "quacks" for medical help—for example, in cases where children suffering from gastroenteritis died because of the parents' reliance on a folk healer, the *Obeah* man, who diagnosed the child as possessed by an evil spirit. Only when the disease was well advanced did such parents take the child to the hospital, too late to save its life. The Georgetown Hospital administration in 1977 planned to start a gastro-clinic hospital to instruct patients about the steps to be taken when gastroenteritis strikes. Defiant and uncooperative parents were warned they could be prosecuted.[6]

Obeah is a term very commonly used among many people of the Republic of Guyana. It refers to the religion of the former slaves. Leon Saul says, "not only was it highly justifiable but there was also the importance of considering a belief in Obeah as basic to the culture of the African slaves." Obeah men have knowledge about both medicinal and poisonous plants. The cultural and religious values of that belief system were eventually recognized as a unifying force among the slaves, tending to make them capable of challenging the authority of the planters. As with priest-healers of other religions, the Obeah men are consulted by people from all walks of life.

Social planners and politicians often attack Obeah as an objectionable and negative force in Guyanese life. If this attempt to "Guyanize" and modernize the culture is to be effective, the program will have to deal with the *Kahimai Puja* of Hinduism and *Cumfa* of Afro-Guyana origin. Anyone working in Guyana has to take into consideration the cultural impact of Obeah on many of its people.[7]

Concern for Proper Health Care

Within recent years, efforts have been made to provide the general population with scientific information concerning health and illness. Some of these concerns have been communicated to the population by radio and newspaper. Most Guyanese do not pay enough attention to the nutrient value of the food they eat, they are told, so they experience decreased resistance to disease and an overall lowering of national health.

The nutrients needed to maintain a healthy body vary from person to person because of differences in age, sex, height, weight, anatomical and physiological make-up, physical activity, and environment. The Guyanese people, unlike the people of well-developed countries, depend on cereal products for about 25 to 50 per cent of their total nutrient consumption. Rice, the major cereal consumed, contains a good amount of protein, while animal foods contribute to iron and calcium sufficiency. Vegetables and fruits provide the A and C vitamins; leguminous plants, especially peas and beans, provide the protein consumption.

In Guyana there are still some problems concerning the relatively few public eating places. Some are not overly concerned with the quality of food served and the conditions under which they serve it. The Georgetown City Public Health Department decided to rank public places in terms of accommodations, quality of food, cleanliness of premises, and related categories. This system consists of letter grades A, B, C and D, from high to low. Each place of public accommodation, including hotels, rooming houses, and restaurants was given a certificate denoting its category. Most of the few eating places were given a B or C category rating, very rarely A or D.

At first, this rating system yielded desired results, since the eating houses tried to maintain their letter grade; but after a while, performance standards began to fall. However, top hotels like the Pegasus and Tower have upheld their high standards. The long lines at Quick Serve, a fast food establishment, also testify to the consistently high quality and good service. Downtown eating houses, however, continue to be the subject of many complaints. Although the prices of food have risen enormously, quality has often spiraled downward.

Health needs of the region were the focal subject of the 11th Biennial Conference of the Caribbean Nurses' Association held August 6, 1978. This meeting concentrated mainly on the important topic of training nurses to meet the complex health problems of the country. Population control and related measures tend to bring new health problems and social problems as well. In these circumstances, said Dr. Sanavitis, nurses have to play a broader role. This view was shared by Rhoda Clarke, president of the Caribbean Nurses' Association, and Miss Walters, matron of Queen Elizabeth Hospital. Edna Tullock asserted that since the training of nurses is patterned after the North American tradition, training should be placed in the hands of Guyanese nurses in hospital settings. In light of these problems, the Caribbean Nurses' Association has endeavored to modify the training since the 12th Biennial Conference.[8]

Another area of concern in health care is the proper care of children of working mothers. There are two day-care centers run by the municipality, one at South Road and the other at La Penitence. The cost for the service has been kept nominal, e.g., 15 cents (Guyana) per day for one child and 25 cents (Guyana) for two children in 1979. The center is open every day except Sunday and holidays, and only children of working mothers are accepted. A nurse is on hand to take care of the youngsters, and, in addition to the city council, UNICEF helps them.[9]

Another aspect of health in which mothers need advice and help is the care and feeding of their babies. A writer for the *Sunday Chronicle* criticized the many mothers who no longer breast-feed their babies. He claimed to know of an infant boy who weighed seven pounds at birth, but after four months, weighed only five pounds. His sister, an eighteen month old baby who weighed twelve pounds dropped to eight pounds within a very short time. Such weight loss, he contended, was due to milk products sold by multinational food companies to both rich and poor mothers. The poor buy the infant formula products but they cannot afford to use the product in the manner prescribed by the instructions, with the result that they dilute the milk product so that it loses its nutritional content. Claiming that they do not have time to nurse their babies, these mothers turned away from breast-feeding their infants. This is not only prevalent in Guyana, but many other regions. The Infant Formula Action Coalition in the U.S.A. took the matter into consideration and urged a boycott of the companies' products. It also cautioned the mothers and tried to convince them not to use these products.[10]

On the whole, the Guyanese people seem to need a drastic change in food production and eating habits. A 1976 survey revealed a 50 per cent iron deficiency in certain sections of the Guyanese population. Another 1976 study showed that every third person suffered from anemia. Whether the anemia is due to malabsorption syndrome or iron-poor food, or whether the problem is related to "sickle-cell anemia," is of concern to scientists working on the problem. The National Science Research Council (NSRC) has been active in research in this area. Research in nutrition among pregnant women resulted in extensive dietary revision, which is going on even today. The Council has several research committees, on medicine, forestry, agriculture, science and industry. The NSRC exercises considerable influence on the nation's health; the Parliament of Guyana has given NSRC official status by law.

William Longgood and Ruth Winter have been working together and speaking out against poisons found in food. They have written two books: *The Poisons in Your Food* and *Beware of the Food You Eat*. They enumerate the sources of chemical contamination from the fertilizers applied to growing food plants up to the time that the agricultural products are eaten. Pesticides seem to be the most dangerous, with their potential to damage an individual's nervous system.[11]

Skim milk is a highly nourishing but often ignored food. Since milk contains most of the vitamins and minerals necessary for good health, it should form an essential part of one's diet. Skim milk has many advantages: it is inexpensive and contains little fat, it prevents stunted growth, and it can be mixed with cereals. pudding, etc., without fear of spoiling the taste.

Dental Care

In Guyana, many villagers of African and East Indian backgrounds use the stem of the black sage tree, which grows wild in the countryside, as a brush for their teeth. They chew one side of the "brush" with their teeth, producing juices which they believe to have a protective effect on the dentine and gums. After the teeth and gums are cleaned, the black sage brush is bent in a semi-circle fashion for scraping the tongue. This daily routine is repeated every morning before breakfast, and the "brush" is thrown away after use.

During the colonial years, many people who lived in the villages and estates would not visit a dentist, even for a needed extraction. They allowed teeth to decay and, as the pain became more intense, they would go to the local drug dispenser (who had no formal training in dentistry) to have the offending tooth or teeth pulled. The dispenser, always called "Doc," would often have a long line of patients, some with swollen jaws, waiting in his drug store. At the back of his shop, he kept a few dental instruments for extracting teeth. He called each patient loudly by name, placed tincture of iodine on any diseased tooth, and warned the patient not to move. At that moment, fear often engulfed the patient so strongly that in many instances he would scream, to be heard by other intimidated patients waiting their turn to be "treated" by the dispenser. Fear so permeated the atmosphere that patients trying to escape their turn in the ancient chair would immediately return home, only to be told by members of the family that they must return to the "doctor." No pain-killing drug was administered. The patient was either seated on a chair or laid on a table. After a diseased tooth was pulled from patients strong enough (or suffering enough) to undergo the ordeal, a glass of salt water was provided to rinse the mouth in the yard. The dispenser then received his shilling (24 cents) from the patient, who was officially sent home, hopefully *never* to return. While the dispenser undoubtedly served a need, at best his services were a primitive exercise of the art of dentistry.

Summary

Taboos and superstitions play a strong part in the cultural traditions of the people. As is to be expected, their influences are much stronger in the villages removed from the urban clusters. The number of scientifically trained health care practitioners has always been woefully inadequate, and their distribution in terms of availability and accessibility to the general population has been even worse. Outside of the two or three more populous cities in the country, obtaining adequate health care has been very difficult. To further complicate the problem, transportation facilities, except for those who live in villages near the coast lands, have always been deficient.

Practitioners of such esoteric arts of *voodoo*, *Obeah* and *poojan* thrive. Many of these folk practitioners acquire a reputation locally for mysterious practices including incantations and supplications to invoke the help of the good spirits and to placate the evil spirits in order to avoid their malevolent arts. The folk specialists, of course, prepare and administer potions for every ill visited upon man. These medications, usually herbs, which, perhaps, have to be gathered at night when the moon is in a certain phase, are then mixed together with other secret ingredients under equally esoteric conditions. People who practice these arts usually boast that their special knowledge is a rich family heritage, carefully guarded and handed down from generation to generation.

8

Changing Health Care in a Changing Guyana

This chapter will focus on selected aspects of health care changes in Guyanese society in relation to some other changes in the basic social institutions, particularly the family. We need to understand the folk background of efforts to cope with illness and threats to health in order to grasp the dynamic interrelationship between social change and the delivery of health care in a developing nation.

At any given moment, the institutional structure of a society may appear to be a static entity; but, viewed over a long period of time, the structure can be observed as a dynamic organization of components constantly changing, growing or decaying. Social change is, of course, a modification in the social organization of a society, and thus it produces a continuous process of subtle variations in social behavior in all societies.

In a rural society social change is typically slow. As each generation succeeds its predecessor, the young move into the positions left vacant by elders. Life continues in very much the same way over generations. Experience is truly the only reliable teacher. In an urban society, social change is more rapid and far-reaching because of such factors as industrialization, education, invention, scientific discovery, and rapid diffusion of ideas.

From the inception of the Industrial Revolution, the pace of social change has increased continuously in Western societies. Multiform change has spread to almost every part of the world, affecting both developed and developing nations to varying degrees. As with the effect of a stone thrown into the center of a placid pool, the surging ripples of sudden unrest move relentlessly across the once tranquil surface. Even the strong family system of Guyana is not immune to the onslaught of social change.

Problems of Families

According to Mr. C. Haynes, Senior Health Visitor at the Municipal Center in Georgetown, the demands of the home are sometimes too pressing and some people escape through separation or divorce. There are many economic, social, and other factors which seem to work against "perfect" family life in Guyana. Officials in the urban areas have enumerated the following factors which are seen not only as causative obstacles to the "perfect" life, but also as the results of a less than ideal family situation:

(1) alcoholism,
(2) the growing number of families headed by women,
(3) young girls becoming pregnant without the prospect of marriage,
(4) the increase in the number of broken homes,
(5) the housing situation,
(6) improper discipline.

While these problems facing the family unit today are certainly a threat, they are not unique to Guyana. Social changes such as the working mother, the day care center, and the single parent are all relatively new to the family structure; they require adjustments on the part of every member of the family. Present in many marriages today are such factors as lack of commitment, irresponsibility, and lack of communication. All of these problems of married couples and families require hard work, cooperation, and understanding to correct them—especially for the children.

Because the child acquires from his or her family an outline of the basic ideology, definitions, and attitudes of the society, the importance of this unit cannot be overemphasized. It is in the family institution that a child's thoughts, perspective, and values are shaped. Today, however, in Guyana, as everywhere, the family seems threatened by individualistic concerns taking precedence over more altruistic orientations. As things appear to be in a constant state of flux, young and old alike lament the fact that nothing is the same for very long. Very briefly, the social functions of the family are: 1) sexual regulation, 2) reproduction, 3) socialization and education of children, 4) emotional/psychological support by love and affection, 5) status definition for children, 6) protection—physical and psychological, 7) religious training, and 8) economic security. In sociology, the term "socialization" is used to describe the ways in which individuals learn the values, beliefs, and roles which underwrite the social system in which they participate.

Family and Sick Role

The sick role, developed in the socialization process, is most important in physical and mental disorders. A patient first learns his sick role at home. He may later be obliged to act it out in a hospital in relation to administrators, physicians, nurses, chaplain, his visiting family, and to other members of society in the manner in which he has internalized this role from infancy.

According to Parsons, there are four aspects to the sick role of a patient: 1) the sick person is exempted from his normal social responsibilities, depending upon the seriousness of the illness; 2) the sick person cannot help himself, and must be cared for by others; 3) the sick role is viewed as a misfortune, hence it is assumed that the sick person will want to get well, and is under an actual obligation to do so; 4) finally, it is the obligation of the sick person to seek competent help, usually from a physician, and to cooperate with the health care professional in getting well.[1] Since Parsons was viewing sick role from an American perspective, it must be recognized that "competent help" in some cultures may reserve a place for the practitioner of folk medicine.

The classic analysis of the way family socializes the individual to the sick role as a function of culture is Zborowski's study on the cultural components of pain.[2] He notes that, in his study of patients from different ethnic backgrounds, Italians considered pain as a physical misery to be complained about, to be relieved immediately, and then forgotten. Jewish patients, from their viewpoint, often regarded pain as something to be complained about, but also to be worried about in relation to its significance for one's future and the future of one's family. "Old American" patients seemed to take a "detached and unemotional view of their symptoms." These "Yankee" and Irish patients viewed pain as something to be endured rather stoically, but to be relieved scientifically and with an optimistic expectation regarding the eventual outcome.

In general, the behavior patterns and attitudes of the sick role are initially formed during the socialization process within the family by the parents' response to the sick child's crying—normally, by appropriate sympathy and concern on the part of the parents. However, an overprotective and worried attitude on the part of the parents may foster more complaints and tears. From this the child may learn to utilize each painful experience and to look for sympathy and help. Thus, it is possible to see how the family, through the socialization process, influences the growing child's definition of sick role behavior in relation to health care.

Family roles of adults can be seriously affected by illness, bringing about a reshaping of roles and role responsibilities. Role reversal between parents can or must occur if the breadwinner's responsibility is switched and patterns of child care may need to change. For example, if a longshoreman loses his leg through an on-the-job accident, he will no longer be able to act out his occupational role since the use of both legs is necessary for him to perform his work successfully. His wife must now become the breadwinner and he becomes the homemaker. Such transitions can be sources of confusion in identity for children during the early developmental stages, especially if there had been prior inadequate role performances on the part of the parents.

The family also influences health and health care through its providing nurture or environment for the individual member. A family of ten crowded into an inadequate home without sufficient heat and enough finances for balanced meals will be more likely to become ill, and the individual's risks to health will reflect his experience of living under such conditions. Membership in a family is a deep and varied root in us all, directing much of our behavior though we may not consiously realize it. It shapes the ways we perceive health and illness and the things we expect from health care.

Serious injury or illness can constitute a crisis even in well-organized families, and its effect is likely to be more traumatic for a disorganized or broken family unit. Such a family is characterized by "dissolution or fracture of a structure of social roles when one or more members fail to perform adequately their role obligations." Examples involve 1) illegitimacy; 2) annulment, separation, divorce, desertion; 3) "empty shell" existence (i. e., living together as a group behind a facade of unity with little communication and emotional support for each other); 4)absence of a spouse because of imprisonment or war; and 5) unwilled major role failure through mental, emotional, or physical illness.[3]

For all of the reasons noted, then, it is wholly justifiable to assert that "the family is the unit of medical care because it is the unit of living."[4] Most obviously, the family is related to health by biological inheritance. Diseases such as sickle cell anemia, RH incompatibility, and tendencies to diabetes, tuberculosis, and poor dentition are examples of entities passed by the family through the gene pool. Heredity is responsible for darker teeth with translucent appearance. These darker teeth lose their enamel more readily than normal teeth and wear down more often to the gum line.[5]

If a father learns that he is a carrier of a disease which affects his children, or if one learns that one is a victim of a disease of a familial nature, this knowledge can bring about complicated emotional problems in family interaction. For example, the birth of a deformed infant may be accompanied by a guilt reaction on the part of one parent or both parents. One can speculate upon the possible emotional distrubances of the family in the specific case of muscular dystrophy, which is carried by the female and attacks the male. The need of a parent to deny knowledge about such discomforting facts is understandable; however, there is a tendency for the parent to believe that certain facts must be disproved and to continually seek other advice in order to get different answers. At this stage of family crisis, there is a great need to see the family as a unit of treatment.

The family, as the most universal of all human institutions, varies widely in structure from the consanguineal (i.e., extended kin groups which include a wide variety of related persons) to the conjugal (consisting simply of an adult couple and their children). The conjugal family acts as a source of "refuge" in mass society—a place where the individual may engage in genuinely personal relationships in a world become largely impersonal.

Family Typology

Various sociologists have stressed that the type of family—based on its values, norms, attitudes, etc.—is more important than its structure. Sorokin, for example, identified three family types: the compulsive, the contractual, and the familistic.[6] In the compulsive family, the bond holding members together is not love but force, and the relationship is based on exploitation, cruelty, and deprivation. The contractual type emphasizes reciprocal profit and advancement to the participants but is relatively devoid of love and hatred. The familistic type is based on mutual love between the spouses and is characterized by devotion, sacrifice, solidarity, sharing, permanence, and stability. Sorokin asserted that the three types of families have been present in all societies, changing in proportion with time; the modal one in today's Western society is contractualism, he concluded.

Knowledge of family type can help us understand the behavior of a patient and members of his family toward the sick person. For example, in severe coronary cases, increasing demands are made on the family to adjust customary routines to the patient's needs. One can expect, therefore, that if the family type is close (familistic) in which each member was concerned about the others prior to the illness, then there will be a greater willingness for members of the family to adjust their roles to help the sick person. On the contrary, if the family type is contractual or compulsive, then the family members will be less willing to make sacrifices to aid the sick person.

Another type of family is the "empty shell" described by Goode.[7] In this kind of family there are no primary group ties such as concern, love, and security for the members. Communication and sharing are at a minimum, so solidarity and permanence are undermined. Each member of this family type is self-seeking; there is very little respect for, or even recognition of, the needs of the other members. As a result, divorce and juvenile delinquency are frequent, especially in a large, urban society. The offspring tend to leave the home of their parents as soon as they can make their own way in soceity; this family type is one which has forfeited virtually all of its functions (except the reproductive) and has, therefore, lost control over its members.

The way in which stress is handled within a family during a sudden crisis will mainly depend upon the type of familial relationships prior to the episode. For example, stress within a family may lead to infectious illness. Research done at the Family Medicine Unit at Harvard Medical School has demonstrated rather clearly that

> common crises such as death of grandparents, a change of residence, a loss of a father's job, and a child's being subjected to unusual pressure, occur four times more frequently in the two week period prior to the appearance of streptococcal infections than in the two weeks afterward.[8]

The same studies have shown that "age, intimacy of contact, and family organization influenced the susceptibility to streptococcal infection." Children of school age were most susceptible and likely to spread the infection to other family members sharing the same bedroom. Chronic family disorganization also was correlated with susceptibility to infection.[9] Additional research demonstrated that "streptococcal and staphylcoccal infections are family disorders, and successful management requires consideration of the family group."[10]

New Times—New Problems

Guyana has another problem in common with some of the developed nations: the problem of drug abuse. Drugs, particularly marijuana, are ever on the increase in Guyana, as measured by the number of offenders brought to court each week. Many Guyanese people believe that such drugs cure them of physical and psychological ills. As a result, at the slightest bit of tension, people are "popping pills." This belief, created in the minds of the people by advertisements, has reached alarming heights. In an attempt to deal effectively with the problem, the Guyana government sent a police officer to Lima, Peru, for a conference on the problems of drugs. Canada and the United States were major participants in the conference.

With this nationwide concern over the use of marijuana, the police department is also on the alert to arrest the people responsible for drug distribution. Psychiatrist Vincent Richards has warned the nation of the impending threat because young students are beginning to use drugs in increasing amounts. Young males who call themselves "Rastas" or Rastafarians, who first attracted attention in Jamaica, are spreading the use of marijuana among young people. The Rastas have become a cult which tries to justify the use of marijuana on various grounds. They say that marijuana is a herb on the face of the earth created by God, and that God did not prohibit the use of it as He had forbidden them to eat pork. Many youngsters are attracted to this philosophy but they do not realize, nor do they understand, the health hazards involved.

There is a school of thought which feels that marijuana should be legalized. However, as in most of the developed nations, officials and most adults are against it. Drugs seem to be imported from Amsterdam, Trinidad, Jamaica, Barbados, and other South American countries. The following solutions have been suggested:

(1) a crackdown of law enforcement authorities on drug dealers,
(2) increased vigilance on the part of the police department,
(3) training of police dogs to uncover drugs,
(4) help on the part of every citizen to eradicate the use of drugs.

Aware that a new approach on mental health is needed, Guyana has applied the preventive approach to this area. Modern socioeconomic stress produces tensions, which it is believed, make people become neurotic or psychotic. To prevent mental illness, employers and others are being asked to provide conditions where there will not be too much strain. The psychiatric clinic in Georgetown Hospital renders helpful service, and psychiatric social workers also visit patients and treat them in their homes. The usual forms of treatment are drugs, electroconvulsive therapy (performed in hospitals), and psychotherapy, very similar to the treatment used in developed countries. The psychiatrist also appears in court when deemed appropriate to give a report on a person's mental condition. The patient cannot leave the clinic until he is certified as normal and able to function. As in developed countries, Guyana, a developing nation, has serious emotional problems of its own.

In addition, the Ministry of Health has tried to educate local manufacturers to guard against possible contamination or adulteration of food products; e.g., preparing ketchup made of squash instead of tomatoes. The Department of Health insists that potentially dangerous drugs (e.g., antibiotics and oral contraceptives) should be bought with a prescription. The Government Analyst Department has stepped up its campaign to bring all drug stores in line with the stipulated regulations. To speed up the process, the Government Analyst Department works in close association with the Registrar and Drugs Inspector of the Pharmacy and Poisons Board. They also seek the cooperation of the Municipality and Public Health Officers in prosecuting offenders. Dr. Woo-Ming has stated that he is trying to establish and enforce higher standards in the handling and preparing of foods.

Facilities and Personnel

It is of interest to note the health care improvements made over the years. The data in Table 1 reported by the Ministry of Health[11] on facilities and personnel in health care depict the type of services rendered to patients across the country.

TABLE 1. *Health Care Facilities and Personnel in Guyana, 1978*

Health Facility	Total	Service Rendered
1. (a) Medical Outpost	13	Provides basic first aid; staffed by Medical Ranger.
(b) Dispensary	29	Provides basic curative care services to the whole population; staffed by sick-nurse/dispenser.
(c) Health Station	88	Provides prenatal and infant care on a weekly or bimonthly basis. Staffed by nurse from Health Center.
(d) Health Center	53	Concerned primarily with the preventive aspects of health, in particular, assessment of nutritional status of children, pregnant women; treatment of minor ailments detected as a result of such assessments; follow-up of chronically ill patients when referred. Staffed by Public Health Nurse.
(e) Cottage Hospital	16	Provides general medical and midwifery services; complicated cases referred to the Regional Hospital. Staffed by full-time medical officer, nurse (midwife), dispenser and sometimes a medical technologist.
(f) Regional Hospital	3	Provides general surgery, medicine, pediatrics, obstetrics, gynecology, opthamology, eyes, nose and throat, X-ray and emergency care.
(g) Special Hospital	5	Leprosy (in process of being converted to a general hospital); psychiatry; tuberculosis (in process fo being converted to a regional general hospital); polio rehabilitation center; institution for aged offering geriatric care.
2. (a) Number of in-patients	51,744	(for all three Regional Hospitals)
(b) Number of out-patients	426,859	(for two Regional Hospitals)
3. Number of doctors	91	
4. Number of nurses	165	Basically trained midwife
	404	Graduate Nurses
	400	Practical Nurses
	177	Nurses Aides
	284	Graduate Nurses with Midwifery
5. Number of Dentists	12	
6. Number of Dental Auxiliaries	12	

Table 1 identifies some impressive advances in an evolving system of health care. The facilities must be staffed and used, thereby creating a need for educated personnel and an aware population—two major strides forward from the folk medicine of the interior.

Furthermore, as evidenced by the subdivisions of care from minor preventive to major curative, one can infer a growing attitude of responsibility for one's own health as opposed to the passive surrender to the mystical components of disease. Rather than waiting for a head cold to develop into a life-threatening case of pneumonia, one can obtain medical help and, in so doing, can assert a sense of control over one's body, in contrast with the position of being at the mercy of unknown forces and the vulnerability of one's body.

Being in the position of control is still a relatively new perspective for the Guyanese. Traced historically, the struggle for personal and national independence was long and hard. Throughout this battle different nations dominated Guyana and, therefore, created an extra-national framework for the social structure. Since it was advantageous to keep the population subservient and dependent, any local attempts at policy and planning were thwarted.

Within recent years large increases have occurred in the number of patients treated and discharged from hospitals. The number, size and private ownership of health facilities across the country have increased greatly, as have the government's efforts to bring about effective preventive health care measures. Speaking at the 1979 Health Week, Georgetown Mayor Cecil Persaud remarked that health care is an ongoing process and a program in which all should become actively involved. The Central Planning Committe in Georgetown advocated that the broad objective should be to create an awareness that conditions in the environment of the home, school, church, and community should be conducive to the health and well-being of the child.

As noted earlier, the first phase of the Georgetown Hospital was built in 1838 and was known as the Seamen's Ward. However, as the hospital's need for more beds became evident, additions were made. Stretching over the southern section of the city and taking up almost two blocks, the name, Seamen's Ward, was changed to the Public Hospital Georgetown. After independence it was renamed Georgetown Hospital. The hospital is run by about 40 doctors and more than 900 nurses.

In the 1970s a study was conducted to determine the needs of the city in terms of a new hospital. It was learned that, because of the Government's Health Program for Rural Guyana, fewer people were traveling to the city for medical attention.

In April of 1980, the Ministry of Health conducted a feasibility study to determine the future needs of Georgetown Hospital following completion of the new emergency unit. According to Carlton Marls, administrator of the hospital, the study took into account the "overcrowding in wards and at the same time. . . . the priority needs of the country's main hospital."

In an address to personnel at the New Amsterdam Technical Institute, Hamilton Green, the Minister of Health, Housing and Labor, stressed the importance of preventive health care rather than a sophisticated hospitalization and medical care system. He asked that administrators and the community give full cooperation to achieve this targeted objective.

Also involved in the national attempt to promote preventive health care are the pharmaceutical and health services. These agencies are joined in the effort to develop preventive health care strategies rather than merely operating on the curative level.

The Sudden Fall of Death and Birth

Whatever the complex factors were that coalesced to produce sharp declines in infectious disease and death among the Guyanese (see tables in Appendix XIV), the evidence of improvements in health and survival is striking. Infant mortality rates of 70+ (i.e., 70+ deaths of each 1,000 live births annually, or a seven per cent death rate for infants in the first year of life) in 1954 and 1955 showed a drop to 61.3 in 1961; it fell still further to 50.5 in 1978, 44 in 1982, and 43 in 1983. Thus, in the span of a single generation of 30 years, infant mortality in Guyana tumbled from 73.6 in 1954 to 43 in 1983—a decline of 41.6 per cent! Parenthetically, it should be noted, infant mortality is probably the best social indicator of general living conditions for a given people. There can be little doubt that the single most important influence in that remarkable change was the pioneering work of Dr. George Giglioli in his battle to eradicate malaria.

During virtually the same period of time, the crude death rate (measuring the number of all deaths per 1,000 persons annually) fell from 12.4 in 1954 to 8 in 1984, a decline of 35.5 per cent. Of all kinds of mortality in a developing country, infant mortality will ordinarily register the greatest impact on the crude death rate, making clear again that "the family is the unit of health care because it is the unit of life."

Meanwhile, the crude birth rate (measuring the number of live births per 1,000 persons annually) fell from 42.9 in 1954 to 28 in 1983, a decline of 34.7 per cent. The "demographic transition" was clearly on track in Guyana.

A Tale of Two Countries

To afford the reader an opportunity to examine and compare some significant rates in Guyana with past demographic trends in a developed country, the United States, Tables 2 and 3 are presented here. Implicit in the common transformation of these societies—and all others—are such causal factors as industrialization, urbanization, education, scientific discovery, improved sanitation and quality of water, changing values, and the inexorable march of ever more preventive and curative health care workers.

Table 2 (A, B, and C) reports on the sharp declines in rates of infant and total mortality for Guyana between the 1950s and the 1980s. Maternal mortality data are too few and too fragmentary to permit any safe conclusions to be drawn. The time stages at which the respective Guyanese rates occurred, approximately speaking, in the United States are listed for these three indicators of mortality change.

As a result of the mortality declines, especially among infants, life expectancy in Guyana reached an average of 66.5 for males and 71.7 for females in the 1975-1980 period. In the United States, life expectancy for males reached 66.7 in 1955, 71.1 for females in 1950. White males attained 66.5 in 1950; white females, 71.9 in 1949. Non-white males achieved a life expectancy of 66.1 in 1981; non-white females, 71.3 in 1974.

TABLE 2. *Comparative Mortality Rates, Guyana and the United States, by Year of Closest Approximation.*

A. INFANT MORTALITY RATE
[Number of Deaths of Infants (under 1 Year of Age) per 1,000 Live Births]
United States[***]

Guyana	Total Population	Whites	Non-Whites
73.6 (1954)[*]	73.3 (1926)	73.5 (1923)	73.8 (1940)
43 (1983)[**]	45.3 (1941)		

[*]Registrar General
[**]*UN Demographic Yearbook 1981*
[***]U.S. Bureau of the Census, *Historical Statistics of the United States, Colonial Times to 1957* (Washington, D.C.: Government Printing Office, 1960). Prior to 1933, for death registration areas only; in 1923 those areas included 38 states; in 1926, 41 states. By 1933, all 48 states reported.

98   Society and Health in Guyana

B. Crude Death Rate
[Number of Deaths (at All Ages) in a Given Year per 1,000 Population at Mid-Year]
United States***

Guyana	Total Population	Whites	Non-Whites
12.4 (1954)*	12.9 (1919)	⎡ 12.4 (1919) ⎤	⎡ 12.4 (1944) ⎤
8 (1984)**	[8.5 (1979)]	White Females	Non-White Females
		⎣ 8.0 (1950) ⎦	⎣ 8.3 (1970) ⎦

*Registrar General
**UN Demographic Yearbook 1981
***Historical Statistics of the United States. Prior to 1933, for death registration areas only; in 1919 those areas included 33 states. Bracketed data from *Statistical Abstract of the United States 1984.*

C. Maternal Mortality Rate
[Number of Deaths of Women from Causes Directly Attributable to Pregnancy or Childbirth per 10,000 live Births in a Given Year]

United States**

Guyana	White Women	Non-White Women
12.0 (1972)*	13.1 (1946)	13.0 (1955)
15.3 (1976)*		

*UN Demographic Yearbook 1981. These data on maternal mortality for 1972 and 1976 only do not indicate a trend, for the actual totals reported are very small. Rates are adjusted from 100,000 to 10,000 live births to make them comparable with U.S. figures.
**Historical Statistics of the United States. Prior to 1933, for death registration areas only.

Table 3 (A and B) provides some information on rapid falls in the Guyanese crude birth rate and ratios of children (under five years of age) to women in the childbearing years (defined as 15 through 49 years in the UN data for Guyana, but 20-44 in the U.S. statistics utilized). Again, some comparative data for the United States are presented with the *caveat* that our early census figures must be regarded with much caution.

For all of their present differences, these two countries, Guyana and the United States, share a history of colonial rule. Each country tells a common story of human suffering and endurance during its tortuous struggle to overcome killing epidemics and baffling diseases. In the theater of its own national life, each has looked forward to a time when it could say, "Death, be not proud!"

TABLE 3. *Comparative Fertility Rates, Guyana and the United States, by Year of Closest Approximation*

A. Crude Birth Rate
(Number of Children Born in a Given Year per 1,000 Population Estimated at Mid-Year)

Guyana	United States**		
	Total	White	Non-White
42.9 (1954)*			
46.5 (1957)*			
44.5 (1962)**	44.3 (1860)	43.3 (1850)	
26.3 (1976)**	27.7 (1920)	26.9 (1920)	35.0 (1920)
28.3 (1978)**			

*Registrar General
**UN Demographic Yearbook 1981
***U.S. Bureau of the Census, *Historical Statistics of the United States, Colonial Times to 1957* (Washington, D.C.: Government Printing Office, 1960). N.B. The earliest Crude Birth Rate data for the Non-White category are for 1920.

B. Children-Women Ratios
Note: UN data for Guyana: Children 0-4 Years of Age to 1,000 Women 15-49 Years
U.S. data: Children 0-4 Years of Age to 1,000 Women 20-44 Years

Guyana*	United States**	
	White Women	Non-White Women
928.4 (1965)	905 (1860)	930 (1890)
760.9 (1968)		
757.7 (1969)		
754.7 (1970)		
634.2 (1974)	631 (1910)	608 (1920)
642.9 (1975)		
580.7 (1980)	604 (1920)	554 (1930)
	587 (1950)	706 (1950)

*UN Demographic Yearbook 1981
**Historical Statistics of the United States.

Summary and Epilogue

In this final chapter we have examined the nature and inevitability of social change (often called modernization) in all societies, whether predominantly rural or urban. The stress of change in contemporary Guyana registers its impact on all institutions, especially the family, since individualistic pressures challenge the older values of self-sacrifice and altruism.

Family and sick role interpretations were considered in the light of ethnic and devlopmental differences, the transmission of cultural and biological links to health and illness, as well as the significance of family structure and typology.

Exemplifying the reality that "the more things change, the more they are the same," Guyana's new concerns about increased drug abuse, mental illness, and food adulteration are signs of *déja vu* in developed countries around the world.

An impressive program of bringing health care to the people is demonstrated by a rich variety of facilities across the country: medical outposts, dispensaries, health stations, health centers, cottage hospitals, regional hospitals, and special hospitals. In addition, there has been a determined effort to expand the numbers of professionals and auxiliaries in the many areas of health care.

These efforts have played a central role in the quiet struggle to improve the level and quality of life for Guyana's people. The cruel waste of young lives, as documented in the high infant mortality data just a generation ago, has been sharply reduced, and more progress can be anticipated in the future. Epidemic and endemic diseases, so long dominating the land and its people, confront new white-coated adversaries in small hamlets and remote villages. Needless pain, suffering, and premature death no longer rule with their customary savagery and fear; they have been challenged and defeated on many fronts, yet others still remain.

There is still much work to do, as the comparative data on developing and developed trends made clear. Sustained and intensive work will continue to be vital to assure future improvements. In addition, it must be realized that levels of living and quality of life ultimately depend on *all* social institutions contributing to the well-being of each person and the common good.

The health care experiences of Guyana recounted here hold many lessons, we believe, for other developing countries. In a broader context, there are lessons for developed countries as well. It is our hope that the first of these lessons to be learned will be a recognition of the vulnerability and interdependence of the human family—all of us sharing a common humanity, dignity, and destiny. Once learned, that lesson should spark our best efforts in care for others that goes well beyond health and illness— well beyond national boundaries.

Appendix I
Geography of Guyana*

Area

215,000 Km² (83,000 square miles).

Population

The estimated total population was 824,000 at the end of December, 1978.
The last census was taken in April, 1970 when the figures were:

Males	Females	Total
347,852	351,996	699,848

Guyana is situated on the northeast coast of the continent of South America with the Atlantic Ocean on the north, Surinam on the east, Brazil on the south and southwest and Venezuela on the west. It lies between 1° and 9° North Latitude and 57° and 61° West Longitude, and extends south to a depth of 720 Km (450 miles).

There is no other English speaking territory on the mainland, the nearest being the island of Trinidad, approximately 400 Km (250 miles) to the northwest.

The length of the Surinam/Guyana boundary is 624 Km (390 miles); the Venezuela/Guyana boundary is 672 Km (420 miles) and the Brazil/Guyana boundary is 1200 Km (750 miles).

Local Time: The meridian of Georgetown, the capital of Guyana, is 58 degrees/09 minutes/55 seconds W.
In practice, however, the Standard Time for Guyana is calculated on the 56 1/2 degrees west longitude, and is 3 hours 45 minutes behind Greenwich Mean Time.

---

* Materials gathered for this text were obtained from *Guyana In Brief*, Guyana National Lithographic Co. Ltd., Guyana, 1979.

Physical Features:

Guyana is divided into four natural regions:

1. The Low Coastal Plain
2. The Hilly Sand and Clay Area
3. The Highland Region
4. The Interior Savannahs

The Coastal Plain

This region, with a seaboard of roughly 432 Km (270 miles), is composed of recent alluvial deposits and varies in width from 16 Km to 64 Km (10 to 40 miles). It is extremely low-lying and areas for 8 Km (5 miles) and more from the coastline are below high tide level, necessitating the maintenance of costly systems of sea defense and drainage. The continental shelf slopes gradually northward for a distance of 128 Km to 160 Km (80 to 100 miles).

Most of the people live on the coastal plain, earning their living in the sugar estates, the rice fields, or working in other areas of agriculture or in the towns and villages.

The Hilly Sand and Clay Area

South of the coastal plain lies Guyana's second natural region, the sand and clay area. Covering about one-quarter of Guyana, it extends from the Pomeroon River inland to the Mazaruni, south to Apoteri, and thence eastward to the Corentyne.

The soil of this area consists of sand and clay deposits. This sandy region is dotted with hills which vary in height from 30.5 m to 122 m (100 to 400 feet). Where the sand has been removed by rain and rivers the soil consists of a reddish sand or of clay.

The sandy soils are covered by valuable forests of Greenheart, Mora, Crabwood, Wallaba and other timbers. The sand and clay region contains another source of wealth—minerals. The main mineral is bauxite which is mined around Linden and Kwakwani.

People live throughout the coastal plain, but in this sand and clay area, the population is concentrated where mining is carried on—e.g., Linden, Ituni, Kwakwani—and where timber is cut—e.g., in the "Bartica Triangle." Other population areas are the missions or reservations for Amerindians, e.g., Orealla, Kalkuni.

The Highland Region

Most of the south and the west of the country consists of forest-covered mountains. The mountain ranges include the Imataka Mountains in the northwest, the Kanuku Mountains which divide the Rupununi Savannahs into two parts: the Sierra Akarai in the south and the Pakaraimas in the western interior, with their highest point in Mount Roraima— 2743.2 m (9,000 feet) above sea level.

Some of the largest gold and diamond fields in Guyana are near the mountain ranges. There are also deposits of manganese (e.g., on the upper Barima and Barama Rivers) and also iron ore (e.g., the Blue Mountains).

The highlands are areas of heavy rainfall. Rain falling in this region collects in streams which run off in all directions to the main rivers. Majestic waterfalls (e.g., Kaieteur) and other types of scenery attract visitors from many countries.

The Interior Savannahs

The savannahs, which are called Rupununi from the main river, are situated in the southwest of Guyana. The forested Kanuku Mountains divide the area into the North Savannahs, 5180 Km² (about 2,000 square miles), and the South Savannahs, 6475 Km² (2,500 square miles).

The North Savannahs are gently rolling grasslands with clumps of trees (called bush islands) in wet areas. The South Savannahs are more hilly. Mountains like Shiriri, Marudi and Bat rise sharply from the general level of the plain.

The Rupununi is cattle country because of the grasslands. In addition, balata is collected from the trees in the mountains, and crops of maize and tobacco are grown in the foothills and in the corrals. Hammocks and leather articles and other artifacts are made by Guyana's indigenous people, the Amerindians, who comprise the major part of the population in this region.

Climate

Guyana has an equatorial climate, its main features being high but variable rainfall, high humidity and a relatively narrow variation in temperature. The climate on the coast is pleasant and healthy for most of the year as the humidity is tempered by a steady sea breeze. The daily average sunshinne is between 6 to 7 hours and the daylight hours range from 11.5 to 12.5 hours. The country lies south of the hurricane belt and is not affected by the hurricanes which periodically sweep over and devastate the Caribbean and Central American regions. The coastal rainfall pattern is fairly well defined with two wet seasons — May to August and November to January — and two dry seasons. However, there is some occasional variation.

Rainfall in the forest region averages about 2.67 m (105 inches), and in the savannah region about 1.53 m (960 inches) with a well defined dry season from October to March.

Temperature on the coastland ranges from 20°C (68°F) to 33.8°C (93°F) with a mean temperature of 26.6°C (80°F) and in the interior region between 18.3°C (65°F) and 39.4°C (103°F) with a mean temperature of 28.3°C (83°F).

Lakes

The chief lakes of the country are situated on the coastland, in the region of Essequibo. They are noteworthy principally for their scenic beauty and also for their value as waterways and water conservancies.

The Tapakuma is situated southwest of Anna Regina. The Quakabuka or Mainstay Lake is a few hundred metres off the Tapakuma. About 19.2 Km (12 miles) south of Auakabuka, are the Capoey and Itiribisci lakes. A remarkable feature of the latter is the existence of a spot near the southern shore where the temperature of the water is evidently higher than that of the surrounding waters.

Gluck Lake on Gluck Island, opposite Rockstone, is about 120 Km (75 miles) up the Essequibo River. Amuku Lake is situated on the west bank of the Rupununi River.

Islands

For over 32 Km (20 miles) from its mouth, the Essequibo River is divided into two main channels by the large flat and fertile islands of Leguan, 47 Km^2 (about 18 square miles), Wakenaam, 44 Km^2 (about 17 square miles) and Hogg Island, 57 Km^2 (about 22 square miles). Fort Island is situated off the middle of Hogg Island, on the eastern side. It is of historical interest for it was the seat of Government of the country during the Dutch colonial era.

Kyk-over-al is situated off Kartabu, at the confluence of the Guyuni and Mazaruni Rivers. From its position, an uninterrupted view over the stream of the Guyuni, Mazaruni and Essequibo Rivers is presented, hence the name which means "See Over All."

On the Demerara River, 24 Km to 33 Km (15 to 20 miles) from the mouth, are the islands of Inver, Borselem and Biesen. At the mouth of Berbice River is Crab Island, while Bird Island is off the Pomeroon Coast.

River System

Guyana has an elaborate system of rivers and creeks. Most of these rivers have their sources in the great mountain ranges of the south and west and flow northerly and easterly, reaching the Atlantic Ocean after meandering through virgin forest of vast resources.

Rivers reaching the Atlantic Ocean (in order of size) together with their tributaries are:

The Essequibo River and its principal tributaries, the Mazaruni, Guyuni, Potaro, Siparuni, Rupununi and Kiyuwini;

The Berbice River and its tributary, the Canje River;

The Barima and its principal tributaries, the Aruku, Kaituma, Anabisi, Whanamaparu and Whenna;

The Waini and its principal tributaries, the Barma, Imotaiand Arawapi;

The Demerara River and its principal tributaries, the Kanuni, Kuliserabo, Madewini, Moblissa, Kara-Kara;

The Amakura River forming a part of the northwestern boundary.

In addition to these, the following smaller rivers also flow into the Atlantic Ocean: the Pomeroon, Moruka, Boerasrie, Mahaica, Mahaicony and Abary.

Besides those which reach the Atlantic Ocean, there are the Takutu River and its tributary, the Ireng or Mahu, which flows from the southwestern limits of the territory. The Takutu flows to the Rio Branco (or Parima), a tributary of the Rio Negro, which flows into the Amazon River.

Principal Cities and Towns

The principal cities are concentrated along the coastal areas. Georgetown, the capital, is at the mouth of the Demerara River on the eastern bank. It is Guyana's principal seaport, center of commerce, and the seat of government. It covers an area of 644.8 hectares (1,612 acres), and has an estimated population of 183,000.

The old Dutch town of New Amsterdam is situated on the eastern bank of the Berbice River. It is of great importance as a harbor. The city covers an area of 274.8 hectares (687 acres) and has an estimated population of 20,000.

Linden is approximately 107.2 Km (67 miles) from Georgetown on the Demerara River. At the end of June 1975, it had an estimated population of 27,000. It includes the town formerly known as Mackenzie, site of the operations of the Guyana Mining Enterprises (Guymine) and the two villages of Wismar and Christianburg. The area of the town is approximately 142.45 Km^2 (55 square miles).

Corriverton is at the mouth of Corentyne River, on the western bank. This river serves as the boundary between Guyana and Surinam. The town extends for about 11.2 Km (7 miles), from the Corentyne River along the Corentyne Highway to within 64 Km (40 miles) of New Amsterdam. The town was established on September 7, 1970 with the union of three village districts. It covers an area of 126.91 Km^2 (49 square miles) and has an estimated population of 10,502.

Language

English is the official and commercial language. Creolese, a sort of patois, is commonly used, especially in the rural areas. Hindi and Urdu, the language of the Hindus and Muslims, respectively, are also spoken.

In the interior sections of the country, however, the majority of Amerindian people speak their own language. There are about nine recognized tribal or district dialects.

Religion

There are three main religions practiced in Guyana: Christianity, Hinduism and Islam. The population census taken in 1960 showed the following percentages, by religion:

Christians	56.7%
Muslims	8.8%
Hindus	33.5%
Not stated	1.0%

Ports

Guyana's principal port is Georgetown, the capital (6°49N;58° 10W). Situated at the mouth of the Demerara River, 4 Km (2 1/4 miles) long, it is located on the right bank of the river. Movement of seagoing traffic is governed by the depth of water over a sand bar, extending 8 Km (five miles) seaward from the mouth of the river. The port is linked by a ferry service to Vreed-en-Hoop on the West Coast.

New Amsterdam (6° 1'N; 57° 28'W), the port of secondary importance, is situated near the end of the seaboard in the Berbice River about 8 Km (five miles) upstream and about 16 Km (10 miles) from the sand bar at the mouth of the Demerara River. Bauxite, the principal commodity, is handled from Everton, 6.4 Km (four miles) beyond New Amsterdam.

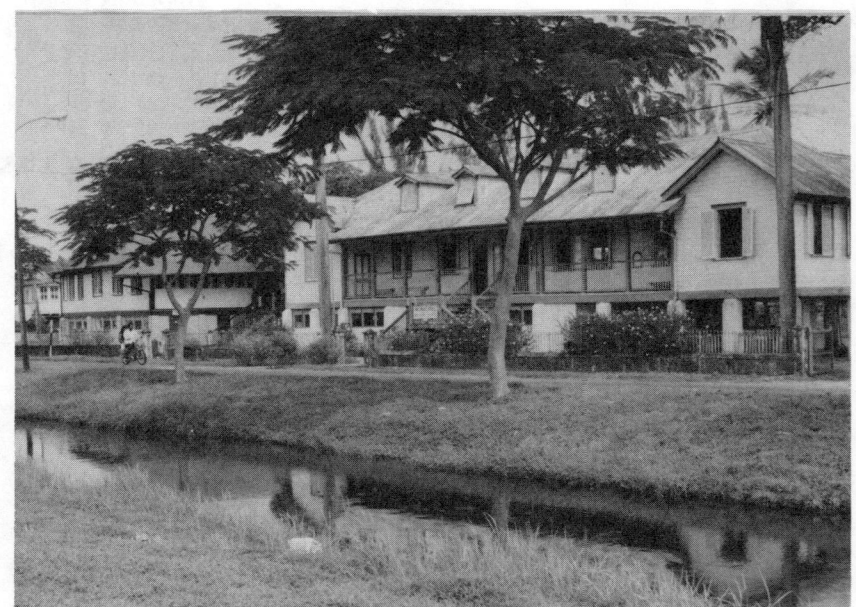

Municipal Day Care Center (Creche), South Road, Georgetown.

Belview Hospital (Private), Georgetown.

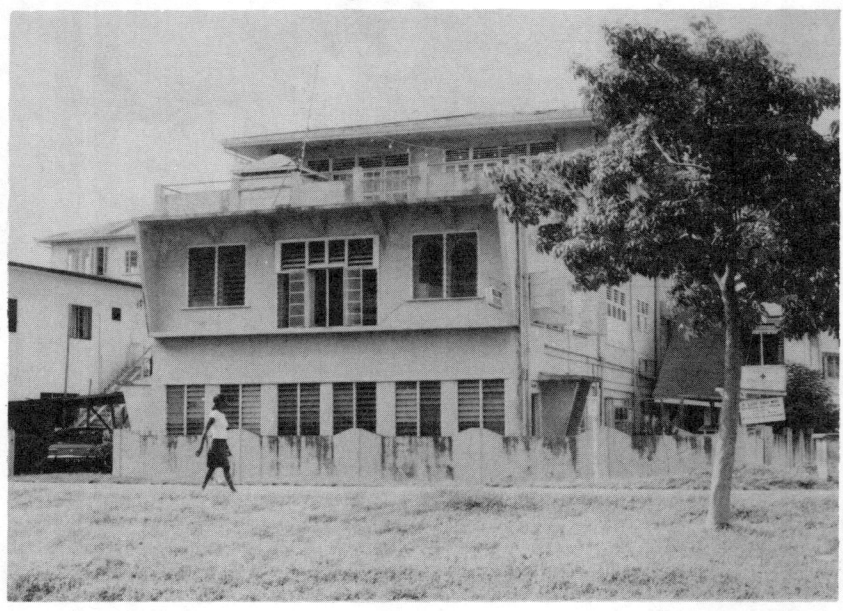

Appendix II
Brief History of Guyana*

Guyana was given its name by the Amerindians who came to this country long before the start of written history. These Amerindians left no historical records and so the details of Guyana's early history are not known. Yet, the Amerindians have left us with the name Guyana, which means "land of many waters"—an expression of the awe which they must have felt as they discovered this river-dissected land. The name also implies the reverence which they felt for the rivers which were for them an important source of food, a major communication system, a source of beauty, grandeur, adventure and the cause of the teeming forests which they inhabited.

It was on the bank of one of Guyana's many rivers that the recorded history of this country started. In 1530, a group of Spaniards attempted to establish a settlement on the Barima River. The Spanish settlement was not permanent. Its ruins were found by later settlers; it must be concluded that for some reason the Spanish decided to exclude Guyana from the Spanish sphere of influence. It was therefore easy for some Dutch traders to establish a trading post on the Barima River. The continued and consistent activity of these traders eventually gained the attention of government officials in Holland; and when in 1621 the Dutch West India Company was created, Essequibo was officially declared a Dutch colony.

The creation of the Dutch West India Company and the declaration of Essequibo as a colony was followed by attempts to maximize the profits from Dutch activity. The system of trade with the Indians gave way eventually to the establishment of the plantations on which sugar, cotton, and coffee were to be the main products. To provide labor on the plantations, slaves were brought from Africa. Thus, the start of offical European colonization in Guyana was followed in less than two decades by the establishment of a system of exploitation based on slavery and the plantation system.

The result of the exploitative European colonial system was that a deliberate policy of underdevelopment was carried on in Guyana. The need to ensure the rigid control of the slaves meant that, though Berbice

---

* Materials gathered for this text were obtained from *Guyana In Brief*, Guyana National Lithographic Co. Ltd., Guyana, 1979.

was colonized from 1627, it became necessary as a result of the limited Dutch manpower for Demerara to be excluded from Dutch colonial activity for a very long time. Indeed, when Demerara was finally peopled in the 1740s, it was necessary for the Dutch administrator to invite British planters from Barbados to participate in this venture.

Even more significant, however, was the fact that, under this exploitative system, the Amerindians, who had been forced into the forests when they sought to escape the necessity of laboring on the plantations, were sought out and encouraged to remain in the forest where they could perform the role of slave-policemen; that is, they were abandoned and restricted to the forest when there were no longer any slaves to be caught. It was not only the Amerindian who suffered in the period after emancipation. The African, who had been dehumanized and repressed while he was a slave, found his effort to develop himself and to make his own contribution to the community to be brutally attacked and frustrated by those who were in control of the society. The Portuguese, Indians, and Chinese were brought in to provide cheap labor under the subhuman conditions of estate life, and in fact, even where some benefited, they did so only through their preparedness to serve the ends which the system determined.

In general, the exploitative conditions of a free but colonial British Guiana ensured that the Amerindians were restricted to the forest; the Africans (after their attempt to become successful provision farmers had been frustrated by the planter group) were restricted to being manual laborers, or semi-professional workers; the Portuguese were restricted to being shopkeepers or clerks; the Indians were restricted to being agricultural laborers and rice farmers; and the Chinese were restricted to being unobtrusive in their ventures. In short, human development was restricted on the basis of a set of ethnic categorizations.

The final result of this policy of underdevelopment was that a number of industries were not started and Guyana's economic potential was never systematically developed. Thus, the rice industry, which Laurens Storm vans Gravesande (Governor of Essequibo) had projected in 1750, was not started until the 1880s. The cotton industry, too, was sacrificed to King Sugar. The forests were never really beneficially exploited, while the mining industry was developed only where it would parallel the structural organization of the plantation. Indeed, where the Dutch confined their activities to the river banks, the British, who assumed continuous control of Guyana from 1796, consistently contained the population on the narrow coastal strip.

In the face of an exploitative policy based on the underdevelopment of economic and human resources, some of those who suffered this exploitation resorted to violent means in an attempt to change the system.

Thus, the slave revolts of 1763 and 1823 were followed by the attacks of the frustrated peasant farmers, which, though initially peaceful (1842 and 1847 strikes) eventually became violent, as in the Angel Gabriel Riots; and also by immigrant disturbances, which, by the 1870s, assumed a degree of violence which led to the Devonshire Castle Riots of 1872.

Even the attempts, by those who suffered, to destroy the system which exploited them were used by the system to create disharmony in the ranks of the exploited. The 1763 Berbice Slave Revolution gave the colonial administrators the opportunity to breed hostility between Amerindians and Africans; the Angel Gabriel Riots were caused by the creation of a system which placed Portuguese and Africans in opposed camps; and the attempts by the immigrants to battle the planters were a means of stirring up hostility between the Indians and the Africans who were the representatives of law and order.

On the whole, however, the masses of people tended to develop strong and permanent links with each other. The villages, from which the main challenges were to come in the post-emancipation period, were communities in which workers of all races settled. The similarities in customs, particularly in the attitude of sharing of goods and services, created a bond among the various ethnic groups which, all in their various ways, based their life styles on a primitive communalism. Indeed, by 1939 when the Royal Commission investigated conditions in the West Indies, the *Voice of Labour* in Guyana demanded the establishment of an economic system which placed stress on the activity of co-operatives.

With independence there came "co-operative socialiam." In 1970 the Co-operative Republic of Guyana was established.

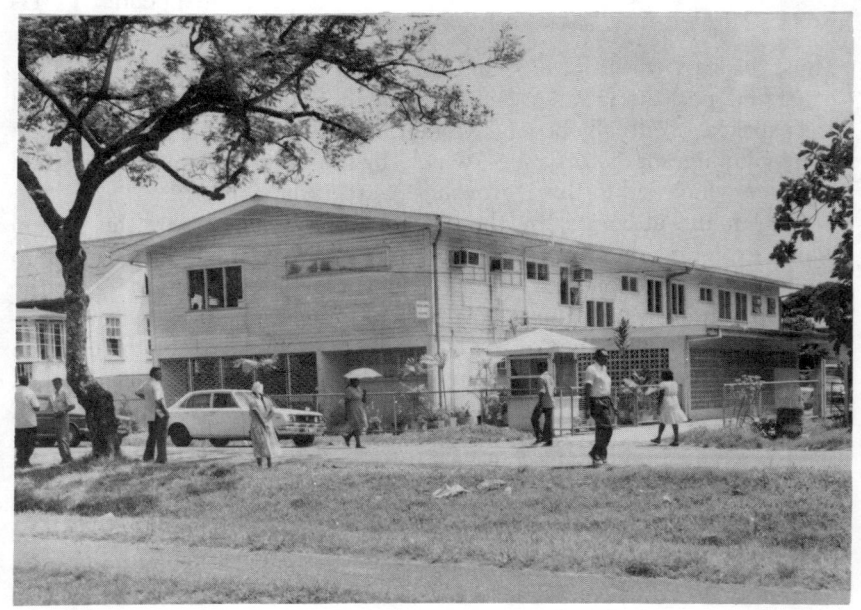

Woodlands Hospital (Private), Carmichael Street, Georgetown.

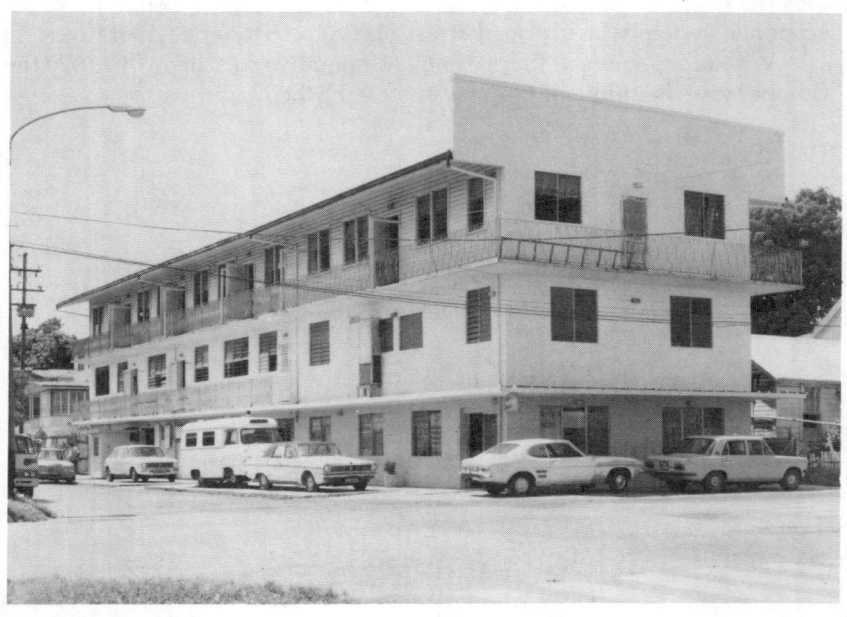

Prashad Hospital (Private), Thomas and Middle Streets, Georgetown.

Appendix III
Amerindians Today*

Spread mainly over three areas of Guyana, the Mazaruni-Potaro, North West and Rupununi Districts, the Amerindian population is comprised of nine tribal groupings throughout the 90 major Amerindian villages to be found in Guyana. The groups are the Carib, Arawak, Wai-Wai, Akawaio, Makushi, Warrau, Wapishiana, Arecuna and Patamona. These are also spoken but not written dialects peculiar to the individual groups, a few of which are common to the various groups. English is taught to the Amerindian school children.

Over the decade 1960 to 1970, the Amerindian population increased by over 8,000 from 25,453 to 34,302 with a significant shift from a prior predominantly male to a current predominantly female population, which augurs well for the future of the Amerindian population. The main reasons for this marked population increase, of course, are the improving health care practices in Amerindian areas and the concomitant declines in mortality (especially among infants and females in the general population).

The three administrative districts, the Mazaruni-Potaro, North West and Rupununi, are the overall responsibility of Hinterland Affairs Officers. Each political unit of the Amerindian society, the village, is headed by a Captain or Touchau elected by the people to maintain law and order in the village. In turn, the Captain, who is paid a monthly stipend by the government, is responsible to the Hinterland Affairs Officer.

Although they exist mainly by hunting, fishing and farming, the Amerindians show a marked trend towards the adoption of a money economy. In forested areas a significant number of men work on the timber grants for several months at a time, while the women and children take care of the farms. Similarly, in the Rupununi, large numbers of Amerindian men work as *vaqueros* on the extensive cattle ranches, which are the mainstay of the district's economy. In the Upper Mazaruni area, site of the future Hydro-electric Project, Amerindians are employed as miners, guides, etc., and are engaged in a variety of other activities associated with the project.

* Materials gathered for this text were obtained from *Guyana In Brief*, Guyana National Lithographic Co. Ltd., Guyana, 1979.

It is said that the Amerindian community is the only one in which unemployment is non-existent among the male working population. Where formerly traditional agriculture was practiced at a subsistence level by the Amerindians, today, with the Government Regional Development System in operation, agricultural crops have been extended from the basic yams, plantains, coconuts and cassavas to include peanuts, blackeye peas, cabbages, and tomatoes for market.

Cassava is still the main Amerindian diet, used in a variety of forms —cassava bread, cassareep, farine (cereal) and cassiri (wine). Pepperpot, made of cassareep, meat and pepper, is a national dish of Guyana, eaten by all cultural groups in society.

The Amerindian contribution to the entire cultural complex of Guyana includes:

(1) Processing of bitter cassava to neutralize its poison
(2) Making and use of hammocks
(3) Identification and use of innumerable medicinally valuable indigenous plants
(4) Manufacture and use of poisons such as curare and wourali
(5) Making and use of fish-catching devices
(6) Manufacture and manipulation of woodskins and dugouts
(7) Training of hunting dogs
(8) Domestication and "education" of the parrot (Amerindians first taught them to speak)
(9) Building and thatching of the benab (one of which is to be found in Georgetown, used for hosting receptions and exhibitions, etc.)
(10) Naming of a large percentage of the country's rivers, mountains, flora and fauna
(11) Use of Warishi for droghing (carrying of heavy loads) in a basket (warishi) on one's back

Many years of contact with other cultures of early missionaries, miners from other parts of Guyana, teachers, etc., have brought about the eradication of an entirely tribal way of life, but the Government's program of training Amerindians to help one another is in itself a fostering of one tribal characteristic—that of co-operativism. Each year, numbers of Amerindians, drawn from the various villages, are given scholarships to secondary schools and technical schools, as well as training in the medical and agricultural fields.

In April 1976, titles to ancestral lands were handed over to Amerindians for collective ownership in keeping with the co-operative socialist spirit of the nation. The lands are owned and worked collectively for the benefit of the Amerindians and the nation as a whole.

Their religion, though Christian to a large extent, has some indigenous practices, and the Macushi, Akawaio and other Carib-speaking tribes have developed a formal religion which they call the Alleluiah religion, incorporating elements from the original Amerindian system of beliefs and rituals.

The Amerindians, though still adhering in some ways to the best of their indigenous cultures, are no different in outlook, hopes or aspirations from the other citizens of Guyana.

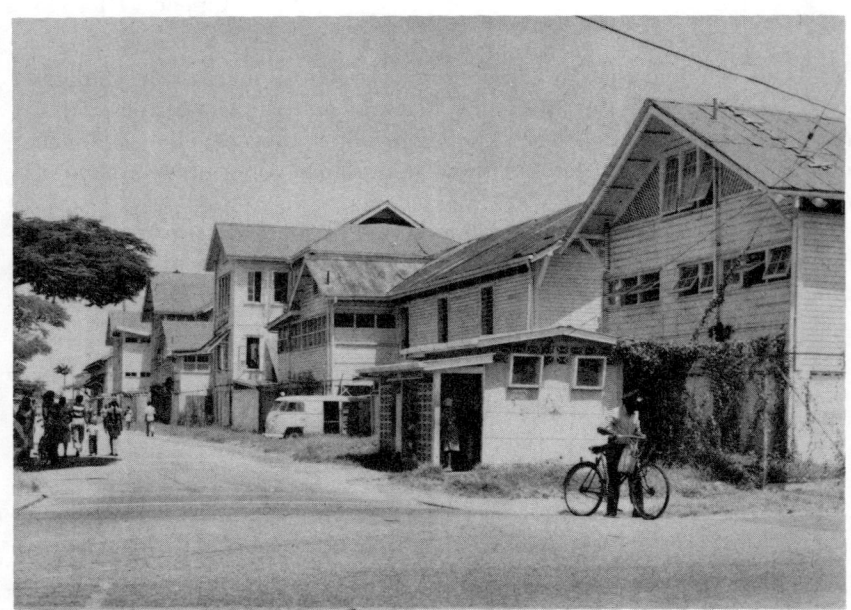

Public Hospital, Georgetown. View from Thomas Street.

Red Cross Convalescent Home for Children, Parade Street, Georgetown.

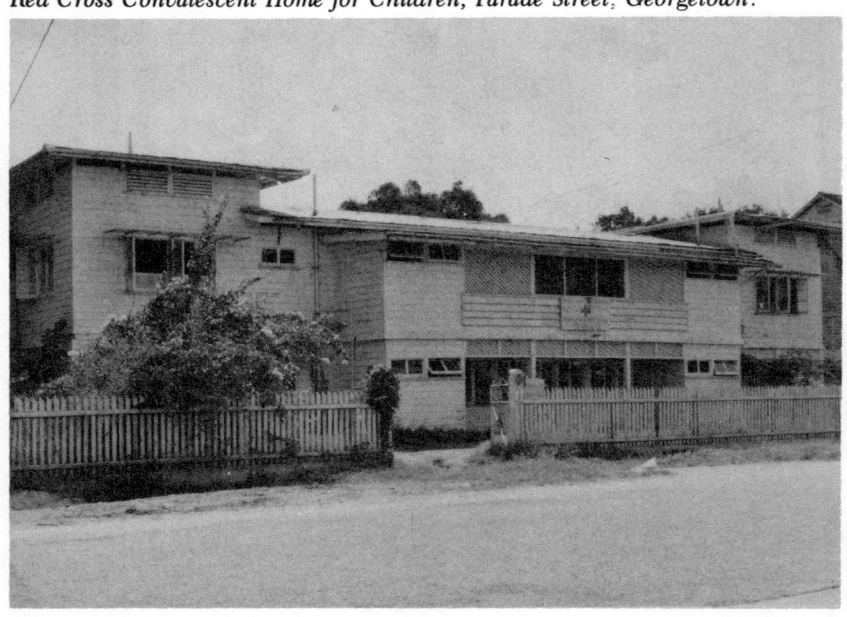

Appendix IV
Constitution of Guyana*

The Constitution provides for a sovereign democratic Republic of Guyana, with a President as Constitutional Head of State. The Constitution provides for the safeguarding of the fundamental freedoms of the individual, irrespective of race, place of origin, political opinions, color, creed or sex. There is a Prime Minister and a Cabinet responsible collectively to the National Assembly, which consists of 53 members elected by secret ballot under a system of proportional representation.

Under this system, seats are awarded to parties strictly in proportion to the percentage of votes cast for each party. The People's National Congress Government fixed the legal voting age at 18; 18 years has also become the age of majority. An Elections Commission has the general direction and supervision of the registration of voters and the conduct of elections. Appointments to the Judicial Service, the Public Service and the Police Service are the responsibility of impartial Commissions.

The most important sections of the Constitution are especially entrenched, amendment requiring the support of a majority of voters in a referendum, or in certain circumstances, a two-thirds majority of all members of the National Assembly.

---

* Materials gathered for this text were obtained from *Guyana In Brief*, Guyana National Lithographic Co. Ltd., Guyana, 1979.

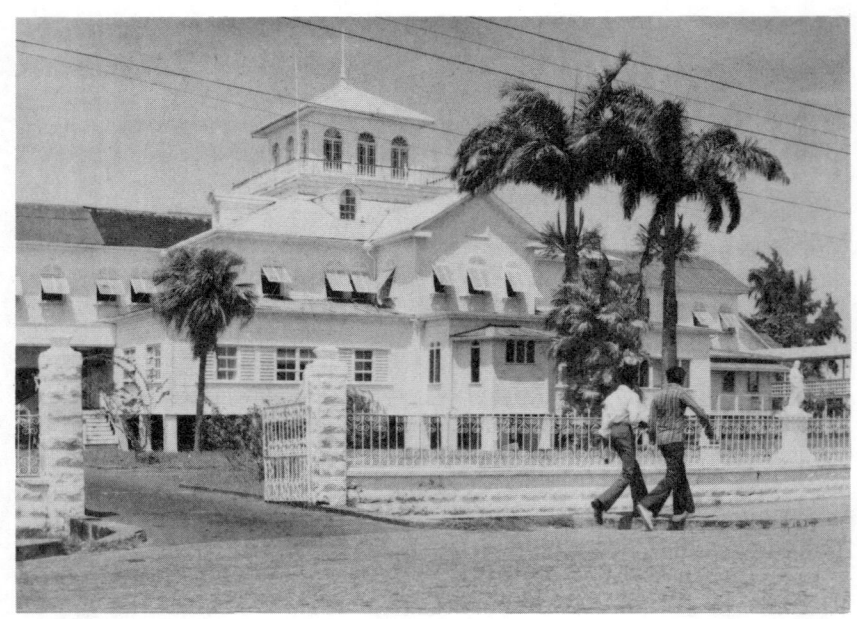

St. Joseph Mercy Hospital, Georgetown.

Medical Arts Center, Thomas Center, Georgetown.

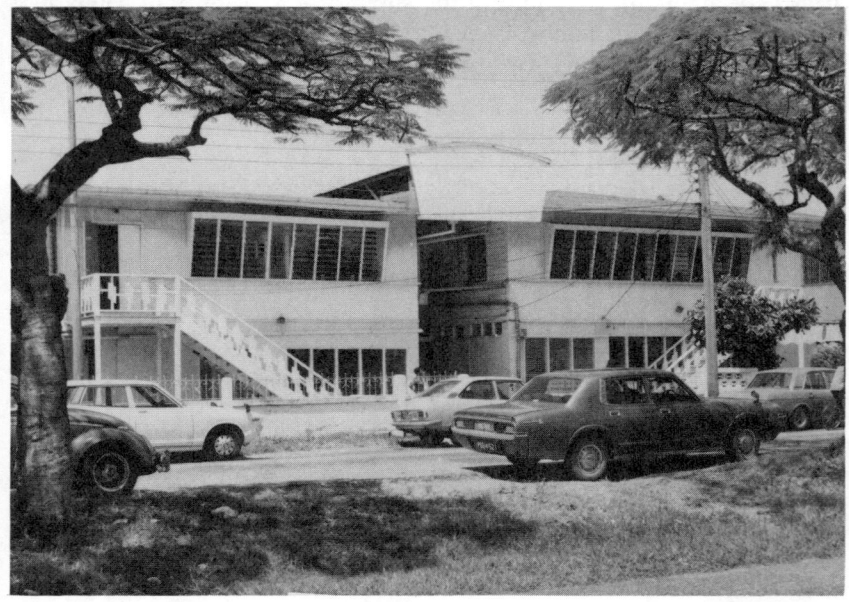

Appendix V
Constituent Assembly*

Following the July 10, 1978 Referendum at which 97.4 per cent of those who voted gave the People's National Congress Government their approval to proceed with constitutional reform for the nation, Parliament resolved itself into a Constituent Assembly by a two-thirds majority vote on November 6, 1978.

The Constituent Assembly is charged with the responsibility of receiving memoranda from the public and taking both oral and written evidence from various individuals and organizations in order to prepare a new constitution for the Republic of Guyana.

It has already begun to do so, and is in receipt of memoranda from various organizations and members of the public. When the new Constitution is written and adopted, it is intended that it reflect the aspirations, objectives and thrust of the people of Guyana, and in effect be written by the people of Guyana.

There is provision for all members of Parliament to be members of the Constituent Assembly but so far the major opposition party, the People's Progressive Party, has boycotted all of its sittings.

* Materials gathered for this text were obtained from *Guyana In Brief*, Guyana National Lithographic Co. Ltd., Guyana, 1979.

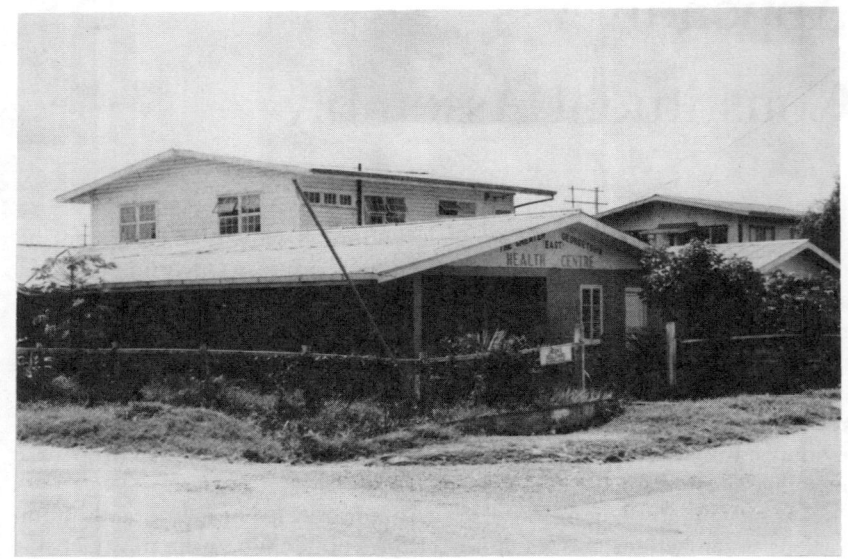
Greater Georgetown (East) Health Center, Campbellville.

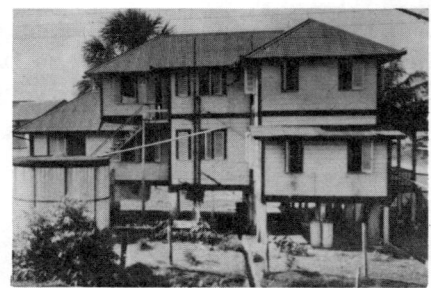
Public Hospital, Bartica, Essequibo.

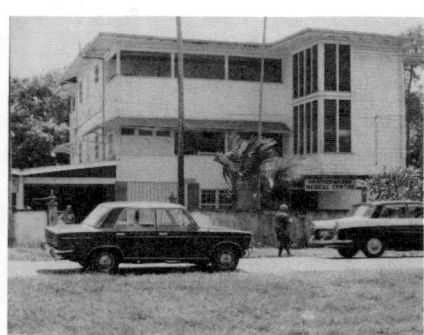
Practitioners Medical Centre (Private), Carmichael Street, Georgetown.

Appendix VI
Guyana's Cultural Heritage*

Unifying diverse cultural groups into a dynamic force for development has been a challenge to all New World developing countries. The young Co-operative Republic of Guyana has been no different. Perhaps in 1966, when a new flag fluttered on Parliament Building and a new Coat of Arms and national Anthem took form, the Guyanese became truly aware of a cultural identity. Immediately, phrases like cultural cross-fertilization, cultural potpourri, and Guyanese cultural identity, were bandied about by all and sundry, some of whom were even calling for a Guyanese language involving creolese expressions. It is not strange that the Guyana Government has successfully used such an atmosphere of national cultural fervor for achieving national unity.

Some years ago a visitor to Guyana may have experienced the strange mixture of religion and joy resulting from ancestral spirit possession in the African Cumfa Dance, or be treated to the sheer oriental beauty of the Hindu Phagwah celebrations or one of the other Indian, Chinese, Amerindian, or Portuguese cultural affairs—Kali-Mai-Puga, a Hindu or Muslim wedding, or maybe Eid-ul-Fitr, or Deepavali, or the Chinese Dragon Dance.

Today, these cultural celebrations have become national legacies. With Phagwah, it is drumbeats, ringing cymbals, the sound of *chowtal* and the throwing of crimson *abeer*. Uniquely, the rhythms of the Cumfa drums and Phagwah music have been blended and incorporated into songs composed and sung by the Guyana National Service militants at Kimbia—the result of an inevitable cross-fertilization. Audiences are now entertained by indigenous beats—Afro-Amerindian, and calypsos with oriental rhythms. The cultural cross-fertilization has not destroyed existing cultural patterns. Many feel that it has served to bring greater understanding among diverse peoples.

Every year the indigenous sects, Jordanites, Shakers and Spiritual Baptists, decked in flowing white gowns and carrying crooks, travel in procession to the Residence of the Prime Minister to bless and rededicate for him the leadership role.

* Materials gathered for this text were obtained from *Guyana In Brief*, Guyana National Lithographic Co. Ltd., Guyana, 1979.

All Guyana becomes involved in the six annual religious celebrations embracing the Muslim, Hindu and Christian religions. The Amerindian celebration "Mashramani," which means "celebration after a co-operative effort" has been infused into the Republic celebrations and is now the biggest and most colorful national cultural affair touching the State's 5,000 communities. From a celebration involving the tribes drinking *cazac* and *parwaree* after a big hunt or co-operative farming endeavor, *Mashramani* has evolved into a national celebration marking the achievements of the Republic as a whole.

National myth, superstition and practices of the people, are allowed to thrive in an atmosphere of cultural tolerance and togetherness. It can be said that culture and national politics merged when the system of co-operativism, practiced by the indigenous Amerindian tribes and later by slaves and indentured peoples on the plantations, was fused into the creation of the Co-operative Republic. Here, the traditional culture of the people became supreme.

Names like Takuba Lodge, Ayaparu Hall, etc., taken from the languages of the Amerindians, are now common on State buildings. Arriving at Timehri International Airport in Guyana, one gets a first view of a national art masterpiece in the form of the Timehri Mural spread across the inner and outer walls of the building. The mural depicts Amerindian symbols and refers to primordial motifs of the early Guyanese people — the Carib, Arawak, Patamona, Makushi, Wai Wai, Akawaio, Wapishiana, Arecuna and Warrau.

Over $1.2 million (Guyana) was spent in 1975 in the development of national culture through drama, art music, literature and dance.

The nation's efforts in hosting the Carribean cultural exposition, CARIFESTA '72, involving 1,500 artists from 30 countries, enabled the Guyanese to see, not only the similarities among Caribbean cultures, but, more importantly, the beauty of their own.

Artists, dancers, folklorists, writers, etc., are giving new interpretations to, and blending, the folklore and the mythology of the land, a dazzling mixture of the Old and New World—the glory of yesterday with the aspirations of today.

The whirling of the Cumfa dancers possessed by ancestral spirits and the revelry of the Phagwah celebrants are today being transformed into dance performances by the national School of Dance. Writers capture the power of the brave pork-knockers as they "run fall topside" and defy the dreaded Bush Dai Dai, Massacuraman, Adopi, and Fairmaid.

There are special elements in the Guyanese tradition, some of which illuminate the continuous process of adaptation of factors in the history and the gradual evolution of a distinctive way of life. Cde. A.J. Seymour,

A.A., one of Guyana's foremost literary figures, in an article on the Co-op Republic in 1970 listed some of these elements: "They include kite-flying on the Seawall on Easter Monday morning, Tadgah and Divali and the queh-queh prenuptial dances in rural areas, black pudding and souse and metagee and pepperpot and curry and garlic pork, the Seawall, and little white wooden houses standing on stilts sometimes in flood water, kokers, trenches, flat enormous skies, greenheart trees towering in the forests, pork-knockers running the falls topside for fabulous diamonds, Kaieteur Falls and Christmas tramping behind steel bands through the streets of the cities, towns and villages, and the members of Parliament in their shirt jacs."

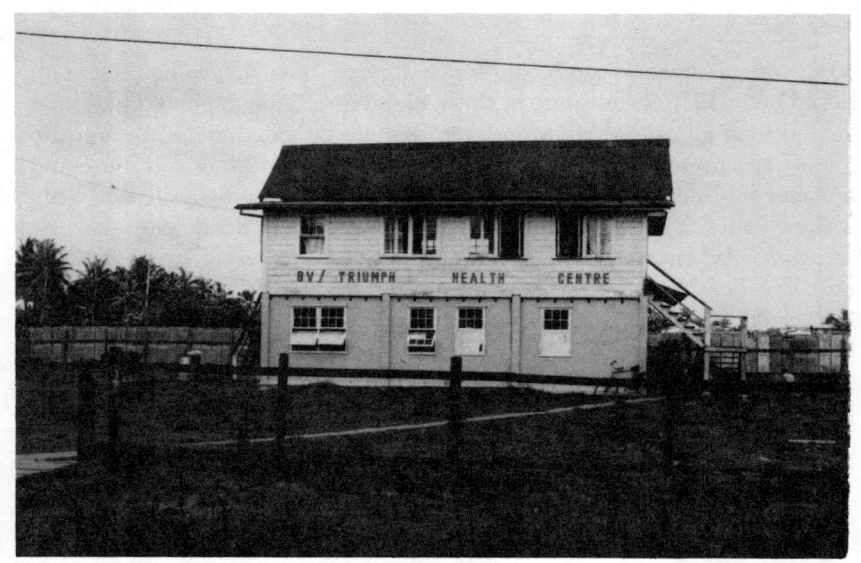

Beterverwagting/Triumph Health Center, Beterverwagting, East Coast, Demerara.

Buxton Friendship Health Complex, Buxton, East Coast, Demerara.

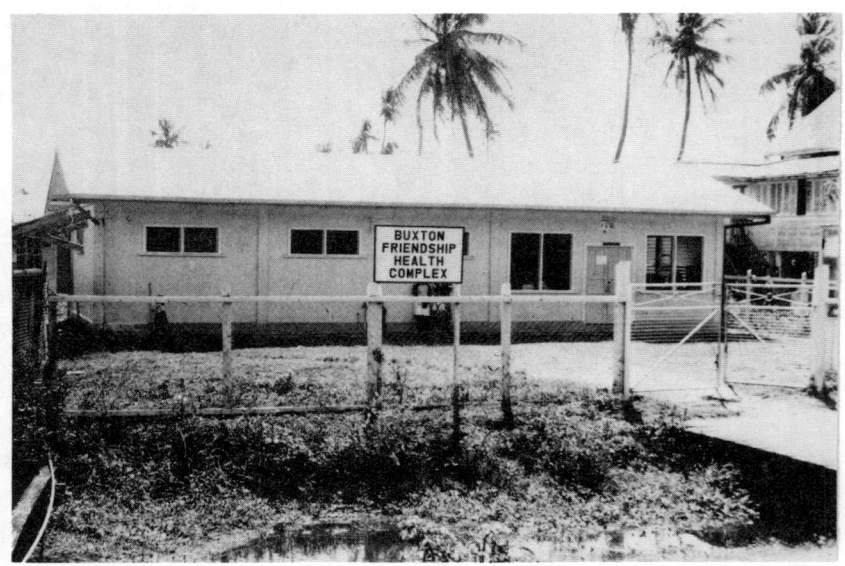

Appendix VII
Religious Festivals*

Phagwah

A joyous Hindu festival celebrating the triumph of good over evil. The despotic King Hiranya Kasipu became so arrogant that he wanted everyone to worship him as God. His son Prince Prahalad refused to do so and was ordered to be burned alive. The Prince was miraculously saved. The festival celebrates the triumph of Prahalad.

You-Man-Nabi

The birth anniversary of the Holy Prophet of Islam, Mohammad. This is also the date on which the Holy Prophet died.

Good Friday

The day on which Christians commemorate the Crucifixion of Christ: a day of solemnity and penitence. Hot cross buns are served.

Easter Monday

The Monday following the joyful festival of Easter Day—the day on which Christians celebrate the resurrection of Christ after his crucifixion and burial on Good Friday. The fact of resurrection is the foundation stone of the Christian religion. Kite flying is an important part of Guyanese Easter celebrations.

Deepavali

The Hindu festival of lights, characterized by the illumination of *diyas* (small earthenware lamps) in homes, electric lights in shops and on public buildings, and fireworks. It is a time of joy, revelry and good fellowship.

* Materials gathered for this text were obtained from *Guyana In Brief*, Guyana National Lithographic Co. Ltd., Guyana, 1979.

The festival is associated with the worship of Lakshmi, the goodness of Light. The lighting of diyas is called "Puja."

Eid-Ul-Azha

Muslim holy day in celebration of the prophet Ibrahim's willingness to sacrifice his son Ishmail on a sacrificial altar. Almighty Allah removed Ishmail just as Ibrahim was about to strike with his knife and substituted a ram instead.

It teaches that Allah will bring peace and happiness to those who make complete submission to his will. In Guyana, Muslims of good financial standing must sacrifice a full grown animal that is free of defect; the meat is shared among relatives, the poor, and the sacrificers' households while the skin must be disposed of in a charitable manner and the bones buried. Meals are prepared late because the sacrifice and distribution takes some time. Sawai—a sweet, noodle casserole—is served on this day. The date is determined annually.

Christmas Day

The day on which Christians commemorate the birth of Christ, the founder of the Christian religion. In Guyana turkey or chicken, baked ham, garlic pork, pepperpot, black cake, sorrel and gingerbread are prepared and shared by all.

Appendix VIII
National Flag of Guyana *

The National Flag of Guyana, the Golden Arrowhead, has five colors —green, gold, red, black and white. The principal colors are green, gold and red.

The flag has the unique design of two triangles (one within the other) issuing from the same base. The outer triangle is gold colored (arrow-shaped) with a narrow border of white along two sides. The inner triangle is red with a narrow strip of black bordering the sides.

The background of the flag is green, representing the agricultural and forested nature of Guyana. The white border represents the rivers and water potential. The golden arrow represents Guyana's mineral wealth and the black border, the endurance that will sustain the forward thrust of Guyanese people. The red of the flag represents the zeal and dynamic nature of the nation-building that lies before the young and independent Guyana.

* Materials gathered for this text were obtained from *Guyana In Brief*, Guyana National Lithographic Co. Ltd., Guyana, 1979.

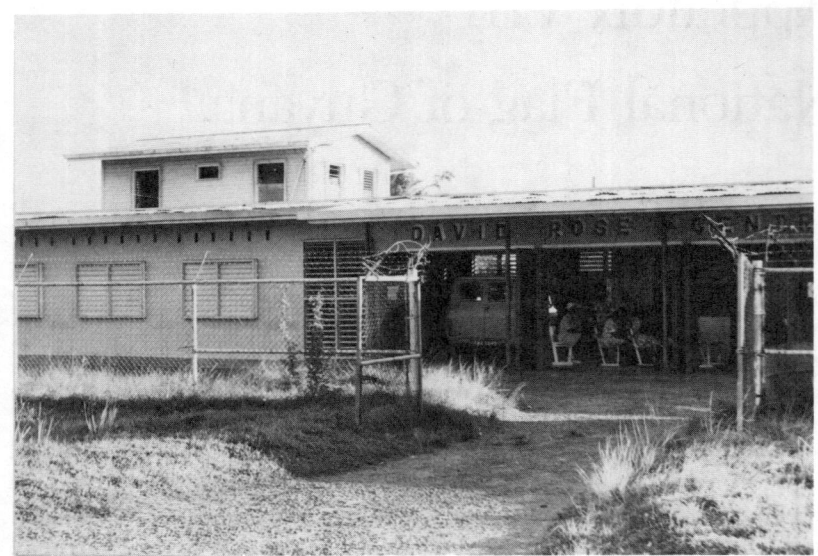

David Rose Center, West Ruimveldt.

Municipal Welfare Center, South Ruimveldt, Greater Georgetown.

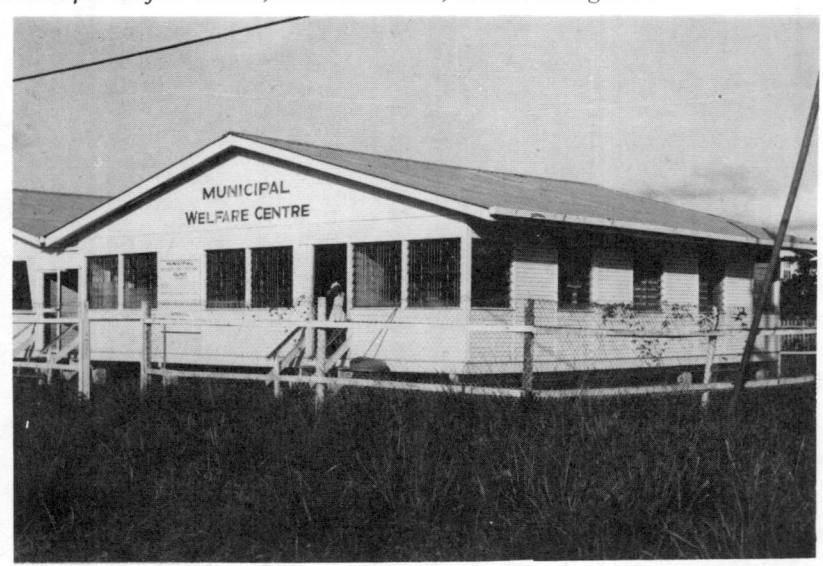

Appendix IX
1980 Budget*

In attempting to achieve a better standard of living for the majority of the population of Guyana, the 1980 budget included a 5 per cent raise for all public service employees, with an investigation pending that these workers may receive a salary that is competitive with those workers in the public sector. Guidelines issued by the government for raises in industry, which has negotiated rates and associated scales, included a 7 per cent ceiling in the bauxite and sugar industries, and a general 5 per cent guideline in the remaining public sector.

In addition to salary increases, there was a 25 per cent increase in personal tax allowance. Incentive schemes were introduced as a stimulus for achieving efficient use of time. Rewards in the form of untaxed revenue can be earned by anyone who meets the standards set for recognition.

An overview of this budget brings an estimated 8-10 per cent increase in take-home pay with a possibility of augmenting one's income (through the incentive program) by as much as 33 1/3 per cent.

*Material for this text gathered from "What the Budget Means to You," *Excerpts from Budget Speech 1980*, Desmond Hoyte, Publication Division, Ministry of Information, Georgetown, Guyana, April, 1980.

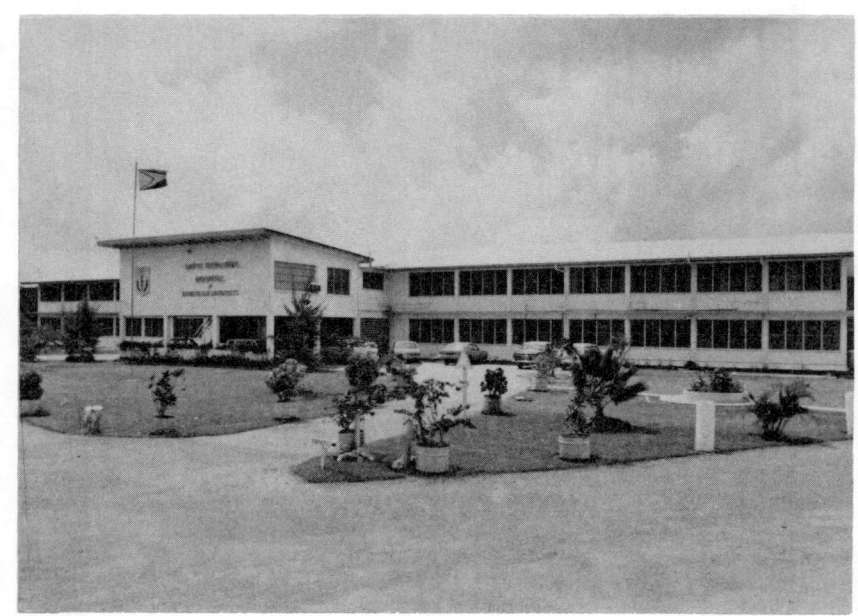
Davis Memorial Hospital (Private), Ruimveldt.

Appendix X
Education in Guyana*

Education in Guyana is compulsory. In 1968 the compulsory minimum age for primary education was raised to five years, nine months. The educational system of Guyana provides free education to Guyanese at all levels in Government owned and controlled schools. The result is that the literacy rate is Guyana is reported to be 86 per cent for both sexes. The various levels of education are:

First Level	Pre-school (Kindergarten)
	Primary Education
Second Level	Secondary Education
	Vocational Education
	Teacher Training
	Special Education
Third Level	University

Education at the First Level

The primary school in Guyana is divided into a) the Preparatory Division, two classes A and B, b) the Lower Division, two classes Standards I and II, c) the Middle Division, two classes Standards III and IV.

The Senior Department is sub-divided into Forms I, II and III, which are parallel to similar forms of the secondary schools.

Promotion from class to class is automatic, but pupils take an annual examination. It takes an average pupil eight years to complete his primary school education.

The Primary Curriculum

The Education Code provides a broad curriculum for the primary school:

1. Mathematics
2. English
3. Social Studies
4. Music
5. Health Education
6. Physical Education
7. Arts and Crafts

* Materials in this appendix were largely drawn from *The Cooperative Republic of Guyana, South America*, published by the Embassy of Guyana, Washington, D.C., 1978.

Besides these subjects, Religious Knowledge, Home Economics, Handicrafts, and School Gardening have been traditionally included in most schools.

Education at the Second Level

The secondary schools lead toward the General Certificate of Education. Government secondary schools, which have a Sixth Form, prepare pupils for the Advanced Level of the G.C.E.; all other schools end at Form V, with the Ordinary Level as the final examination.

It takes an average pupil five years to reach the "O" Level and an additional two years to attain the "A" Level. The subjects taught in the secondary school to the examination level include English, English Literature, French, Art, Spanish, Chemistry, Biology, Physics, General Science, Economics, Pure and Applied Mathematics, Geography, and History. Home Economics and Commercial Subjects are new additions to the curriculum.

Multilateral Schools

Another system of secondary education is the multilateral system. The program of these schools includes five years of secondary education for students between the ages of 10 and 18. Students take a basic three-year course in English and Modern Languages, Mathematics, General Studies, Agriculture, Social Studies, Arts and Crafts, Wood and Metal Work, Home Economics and Nutrition, Music and Physical Education.

With such a range of studies, the multilateral schools are intended to offer Guyanese youth a wide mixture of academic and vocational opportunities. During their fourth year in the schools, the students choose from Science, Technology, Agriculture, Home Economics or Commerce for major study.

Attendance at Primary and Secondary Schools

Pupils attend school five hours each day from Monday through Friday. Classes normally commence at 8:30 a.m. with lunchtime recess at 11:30 a.m. and resume at 1:00 p.m. to end at 3:00 p.m. In the secondary school there are 40 periods, 8 a day, of 40 minutes duration.

The school year begins in September and ends in August. It is divided into three terms of 13 weeks each: Christmas Term—September to December with two weeks' vacation; Easter Term—January to April with two weeks' vacation; and August Term—April to July with six weeks' vacation. A school year has approximately 189 days.

Administration of Primary and Secondary Schools

Internal administration of these schools is effected by the Headmaster and the Senior Masters. The Headmaster is responsible to the District Education Officer for professional matters and to the School Manager for administrative matters, e.g., school holidays, leave of absence of teachers, etc. In most cases the same person serves as School Manager and District Education Officer.

Community High Schools

This system of education is designed to improve the secondary school education offered for students over 12 years of age. One school in each area is designated a post-primary school with the other schools serving as feeder schools.

The program is designed to prepare students for life in the Guyanese society by developing in them practical skills to make them employable for a variety of jobs required by the society. Students undergo a four-year program. During the first two years, they are exposed to basic academic studies, i.e., English, Mathematics, Science, Social Studies, Health and Physical Education, Music, prevocational subjects such as Arts and Crafts, Agriculture, Home Economics, Industrial Arts, and vocational activities to serve the community.

As students are guided through the first two-year phase, their aptitudes, interests and abilities are identified. In the final two years, emphasis is placed on vocational activities while basic academic studies continue to be an important part of the school experience. Based on their ability, interest and aptitude, students are guided by teachers to select a vocational area in which they will concentrate, e.g., Agriculture, Arts and Crafts, Home Economics or Industrial Arts.

Vital to the second period is exposure to actual job experiences and tasks to prepare students for their working lives.

New Caribbean Exams

Since 1978 students have not taken the Preliminary Certificate of Examination (P.C.E.) and the College of Preceptors Examination (C.P.E.). These were replaced by the Secondary School Entrance Examination (S.S.E.E.), formerly the Common Entrance Examination, the Secondary Schools Proficiency Examination (S.S.P.E.), and the General Certificate of Education Examination (G.C.E.).

Students from Guyana and several other Caribbean countries have treated five subjects since 1979 in the regionally oriented exams, replacing the London General Certificate of Education Exam. The five subjects are English, Mathematics, Geography, Caribbean History and Integrated Science. In addition to the exam in these subjects, students can also take the G.C.E. exams.

Vocational Education

There are two vocational schools under the control of the Ministry of Education: the Government Technical Institute and the Carnegie School of Home Economics. Two other Government vocational schools—the Guyana School of Agriculture under the Ministry of Agriculture and the Industrial Training Centre—are under the Ministry of Labour. Two corporations also manage Trade Schools to provide technical training for their respective industries.

The Government Technical Institute offers both trade and technical courses. These include Plumbing, Radio/Electronic Service, Fitting and Machinery, Motor Vehicle Mechanics, Agricultural Mechanics, Welding, Building Trades and Construction, Commercial Education and special courses.

The Carnegie School of Home Economics trains young men and women between the ages of 15 and 18 in Household Management, which includes Cookery and Nutrition, Arts and Crafts, Needlework and Dressmaking.

Teacher Education

There are three teacher-training institutions in Guyana which provide pre-service training for primary school teachers and lower-form secondary school teachers, post-graduate diploma courses for teachers at both primary and secondary levels, and a one year Certificate in Education course for trained teachers.

The teacher training institutions are the Cyril Potter College of Education, the Lilian Dewar College of Education, and the University of Guyana.

Special Education

The Thomas Lands School (for Handicapped Children) is divided into three sections—Oral, Retarded, and Blind—and provides normal primary education for these children.

Education at The Third Level

The University of Guyana provides higher education in the fields of Arts, Natural Science, Social Science, Education and Technology. There are also additional classes in Public Administration, Medical Technology and Social Work. There is also a one year Part One course for law students who are then admitted to the Faculty of Law at the University of the West Indies to complete their degrees.

Minimum admission to the degree course is five subjects at the G.C.E. Ordinary Level including English and Pure Mathematics. The course is of four years' duration.

Adult Education

Adult education is administered by the Adult Education Association with grants-in-aid from the Education Ministry. The A.E.A. provides "upgrading-of-skills" training and orientation in addition to "O" and "A" level classes leading to the General Certificate of Education.

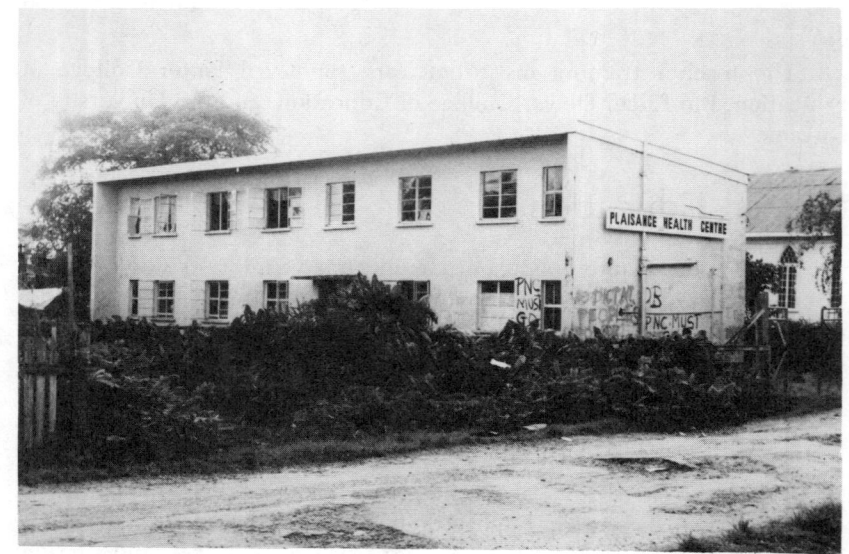

Plaisance Health Center, Plaisance, East Coast, Demerara.

Nabacalis Health Center, East Coast, Demerara.

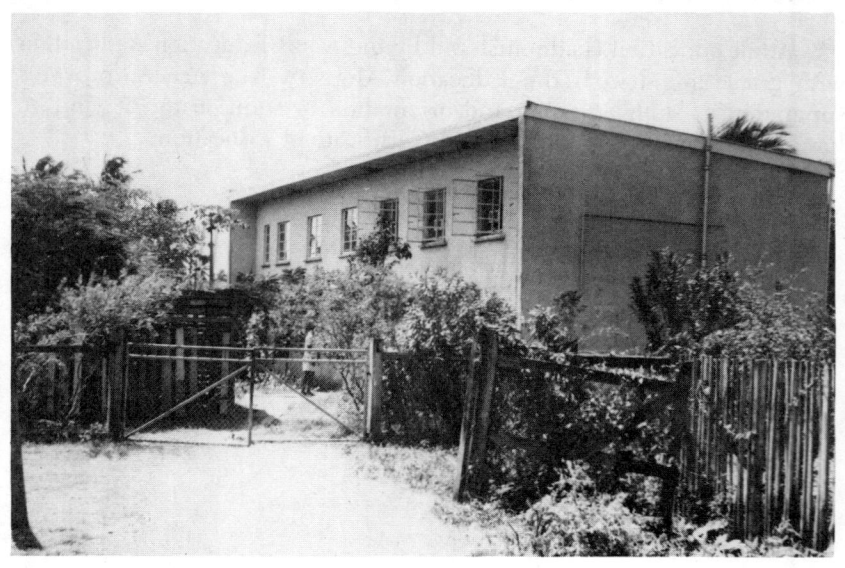

Appendix XI
Major Industries in Guyana*

Milling of sugar and rice and bauxite mining are the major industries of this young nation. The production of bauxite in Guyana started in 1916, seven years after the discovery of the electrolytic process for the extraction of aluminum from bauxite. Bauxite operations prior to 1971 were carried out by the Demerara Bauxite Company and the Reynolds Metal Company. In pursuit of Guyana's policy of national ownership and control of the resources of the country, the assets of the Demerara Bauxite Company and Reynolds Metal Company were nationalized through purchase by the state in 1971 and 1975, respectively. On October 1, 1977, these two bauxite companies merged to form Guymine—Guyana Mining Enterprise, Limited. Guyana is one of the world's five largest producers of bauxite and the supplier of 90% of the world's supply of calcined bauxite.

Sugar, the chief agricultural industry, is cultivated on the coastal area of this 83,000 square mile country—Guyana's narrow coastal belt is one of the few regions of the world where sugar cane can be harvested twice a year. The assets of the Booker McConnell Holdings were nationalized by purchase, on May 26, 1976. They are now handled by GUYSUCO, the Guyana Sugar Corporation, Limited.

It is estimated that 150,000 people derive their livelihood from the sugar industry, the majority being employees of the several sugar companies in operation here. Peasant cane farming is also being encouraged and is yearly increasing its contribution to total sugar production. During 1974 the sugar industry performed creditably, increasing its production by 25% with an output of 340,815 tons. In keeping with its policy of nonalignment, Guyana trades her sugar on a wide international market.

The cultivation of rice in Guyana started sometime around the eighteenth century. The introduction of immigrants from India to provide indentured labor accelerated the development of the rice industry, since the immigrants were accustomed to growing and eating rice in their former homeland. Rice is the staple diet of Guyanese menus.

---

*Materials in this appendix were compiled by *The American Women's Group*, Guyana, South America, 1976.

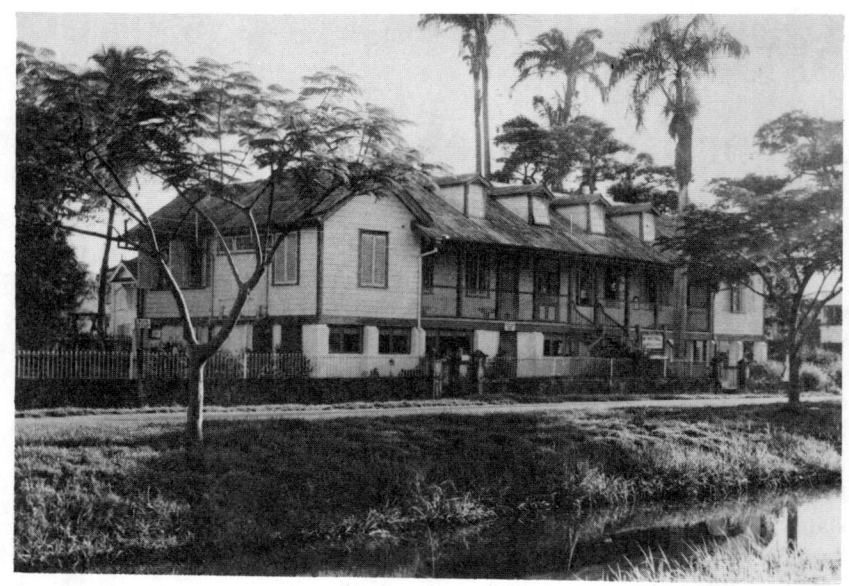

Municipal Day Care Center, side view (Creche), South Road, Georgetown.

Lodge Public Health Maternity and Child Care Clinics, Lodge Hadfield Street, Georgetown.

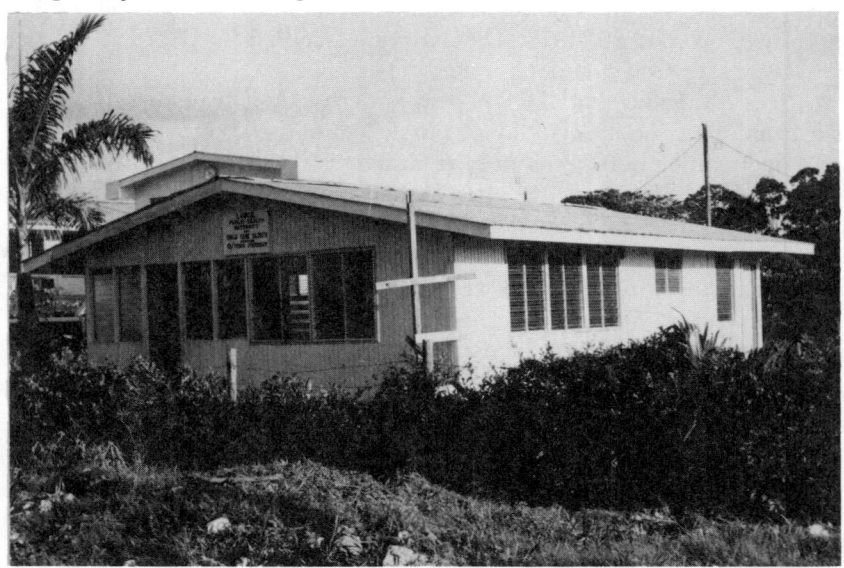

Appendix XII
Local Substitutes for Foods Unavailable In Guyana*

1. Grated raw pumpkin for grated raw carrots.
2. Breadfruit or white yams for potato salad or mashed potatoes.
3. Breadfruit or cassavas for French fried potatoes.
4. Yams for baked potatoes.
5. Green mangoes or green pawpaws in the fillings for apple pies.
6. Cashew apples for raw apples in Waldorf salads.
7. Local dried fruits for prunes and currants.
8. Toasted cassava bread for potato or corn chips.
9. Bora beans for green string beans. (Bora beans should not be composed with bara split peas.)
10. Grated green pawpaw for cabbage.
11. Chilled evaporated milk for whipped cream.
12. Breadnuts for chestnuts.
13. Peanuts for walnuts.

Appendix XIII
Health Facilities in Administrative Districts*

ESSEQUIBO
ADMINISTRATIVE DISTRICT

Description of Area	Estimated Population	District Hospitals No.	District Hospitals Location	Cottage Hospitals No.	Cottage Hospitals Location	Health Dispensaries No.	Health Dispensaries Location	Maternity And Centers No.	Maternity And Centers Location	Child Welfare Clinics
Pomeroon River, both banks from mouth to Pickersgill, including Akawinni River and eastwards along the coast to, and including, Paradise	7,299			1	Charity	1	Charity	2	Charity Pomeroon	3
Walton Hall to Unu Creek inclusive	13,291					1	Anna Regina Windsor Castle Queenstown	3	Anna Regina	4
Unu Creek to Supenaam River and including Tiger Island	9,139	1	Suddie			1	Supenaam	1	Huist-Dieren	2
Totals	29,729	1		1		3		6		9

* Reprinted from British Guiana (Guyana) Development Programme (1966-1972), The Government Printery, Georgetown, British Guiana.

ESSEQUIBO ISLANDS
ADMINISTRATIVE DISTRICT

Description of Areas	Estimated Population	District Hospitals		Cottage Hospitals		Dispensaries		Health Centers		Maternity and Child Welfare Clinics
		No.	Location	No.	Location	No.	Location	No.	Location	
Wakenaam, with Ct. Troolie, Karaburu, Potaroro and Jockey Islands and left bank, Essequibo River, to Anawarri River	7,588					1	Wakenaam			4
Leguan with Hog, Little Trollie, Liberty, Akurikuri and Rock Islands and left bank, Essequibo River, between Arawarri and Groete Rivers	6,582			1	Leguan					5
Totals	14,170	—		1		1		—		9

Appendix XIII

EAST DEMERARA
ADMINISTRATIVE DISTRICT

Description of Areas	Estimated Population	District Hospitals		Cottage Hospitals		Dispensaries		Health Centers		Maternity and Child Welfare Clinics
		No.	Location	No.	Location	No.	Location	No.	Location	
Madeqini Creek (excluding Atkinson Field) East Bank, Demerara River, to and including Houston (i.e., to the southern boundary of Urban Greater Georgetown	22,870					1	Soesdyke	2	Soesdyke Craig	9
Sophia, (i.e., eastern boundary or Urban Greater Georgetown) to Lusignan inclusive	30,998							2	Plaisance Beterverwagting	2
Buxton to Huntley left bank, Mahaica River, inclusive and including Cane Grove—La Bonne Mere Land Settlement	39,186							4	Buxton Golden Grove-Nabaclia Clonbrook-Arms Grove Mahaica	4
Mahaica River to Abary River	10,961			1	Mahaicony			1	Handsom Tree	8
Totals	104,015		—	1		1		9		23

WEST DEMERARA
ADMINISTRATIVE DISTRICT

Description of Areas	Estimated Population	District Hospitals		Cottage Hospitals		Dispensaries		Health Centers		Maternity and Child Welfare Clinics
		No.	Location	No.	Location	No.	Location	No.	Location	
Itaka, right bank, Essequibo River, to Uitvlugt inclusive and including Fort and other Islands in the vicinity	17,099					1	Parika	1	Vergenoegen	2
Stewartville to Schoon Ord. inclusive	25,550			1	Leonora			3	Vreed-en-Hoop Windsor Forest	
La Grange to Kamuni Creek	19,083					2	No. 162 Canals Polder	2	Den Amstel Good Intention Sisters	3
									La Grange	
Totals	61,732	—		1		3		6		5

EAST BERBICE
ADMINISTRATIVE DISTRICT

Description of Areas	Estimated Population	District Hospitals		Cottage Hospitals		Dispensaries		Health Centers		Maternity and Child Welfare Clinics
		No.	Location	No.	Location	No.	Location	No.	Location	
Right Bank, Berbice River, inclusive of Mara to New Amsterdam, municipal boundary north of Providence and to left bank, Canje River, from Greek Lands (N/A Water Path) to proposed municipal boundary of Smythfield	6,655					1	Schepnoed			
Right bank, Canje River, from Vriedenrrienschaup (Port Mourant Water Path) to mouth of river and along coast to Borlam inclusive	16,585	1	Port Mourant					2	Bohemia Cumberland	
Gibraltar to Johns (Port Mourant) inclusive	27,481							2	Fyrish Williamsburg	2
Bloomfield to No. 51 inclusive Blocks I & II	19,517	1	Skeldon					1	Bushlot	
No. 52 to Moleson Creek	25,788							3	Crabwood Creek No. 64 No. 79	2
Totals	96,026	2		—		1		8		4

Appendix XIII 145

146 Appendix XIII

WEST BERBICE
ADMINISTRATIVE DISTRICT

Description of Areas	Estimated Population	District Hospitals		Cottage Hospitals		Dispensaries		Health Centers		Maternity and Child Welfare Clinics
		No.	Location	No.	Location	No.	Location	No.	Location	
Abary River to Zuigwyck left bank, Berbice River	26,524							4	Woodley Park Litchfield Fort Wellington Bushlot	6
Totals	26,524	—		—		—		4		6

MEDICAL FACILITIES IN THE INTERIOR

Hospitals:
    1. Mabaruma (North-West)
    2. Lethem (Rupununi)

Medical Outposts: (Dispenser and Midwife: Accommodation of six to eight beds)
    1. Madhai (Potaro)
    2. Kamarang (Mazaruni)
    3. Acquero (Moruca, North-West)

Dispensing: Annai (Rupununi)
There is a travelling dispenser who runs all the riverain areas in the North-West. The dispenser at Madhai travels around the Mazaruni District.

Appendix XIV
Fertility, Mortality and Morbidity Trends

TABLE 1. Crude Death, Crude Birth, and Infant Mortality Rates, 1954-1984.

Year	Crude Birth Rate per 1000 Population	Crude Death Rate per 1000 Population	Infant Mortality Rate per 1000 Live Births
*1954	42.9	12.4	73.6
1955	43.2	11.9	70.3
1956	42.3	11.2	68.8
1957	46.5	11.2	67.6
1958	43.8	10.0	61.2
1959	44.5	10.0	57.2
1960	43.1	9.6	61.3
1961	43.0	9.2	52.6
1962	42.2	8.6	...
1963	42.0	7.8	...
1964	40.3	7.9	...
**1962	44.5	...	...
1963	44.2	...	...
1964	42.5	...	...
1965	41.9	...	...
1966	41.6	...	...
1967	35.9	...	...
1968	35.5	...	...
1969	31.9	...	...
1970	33.4	...	...
1971	31.7	...	...
1972	33.9	...	...
1973	31.9	...	...
1976	26.3	...	...
1978	28.3	7.3	50.5
1975-1980			47.9

Year	Crude Birth Rate per 1000 Population	Crude Death Rate per 1000 Population	Infant Mortality Rate per 1000 Live Births
***1975	27	7	50
1982	28	7	44
1983	28	7	43
1984	28	8	43

*1954-1964 data reprinted from *British Guiana (Guyana) Development Programme (1966-1972)*. The Government Printery, Georgetown, British Guiana. Source: Registrar General.

**1962-1980 data are drawn from *UN Demographic Yearbook 1981*

***1975-1984 data are drawn from Population Reference Bureau's *World Population Fact Sheet*. It depends heavily on UN data and estimates. Data need not match year of publication.

TABLE 2. Reported Malaria Cases from the Interior, 1960-1964

Year	Cases from Interior	Per Cent of Total Reported
1960	676	100.0
1961	148	62.9
1962	338	95.2
1963	485	97.9
1964	222	98.7

Source: Registrar General

TABLE 3. Notified Cases and Deaths from Pulmonary Tuberculosis, 1952-1961

	1952	1953	1954	1955	1956	1957	1958	1959	1960	1961
Notified Cases	268	283	216	207	196	189	202	170	199	192
Rate per 100,000	59.2	60.8	45.1	42.0	38.6	36.1	37.4	30.4	34.6	32.5
Deaths	168	147	117	124	107	137	77	69	41	45
Tuberculosis Death Rate per 100,000 Population	57	32	24	25	21	26.2	14.2	12.3	7.1	7.6

Source: Registrar General

TABLE 4. Typhoid, Dysentery, and Gastro-Enteritis: Deaths Resulting from Parasitic Water, Food, and Milk-Bone Diseases, by Age Group, 1957-1961

Year	Total	Age Group				
		0-1*	1-4	5-19	15-44	45+
				Typhoid		
1957	32	..	..	10	18	4
1958	20	..	1	5	10	4
1959	23	2	4	6	8	3
1960	14	2	3	..	7	2
1961	20	..	5	1	11	3
				Dysentery		
1957	29	16	5	..	2	6
1958	13	5	4	..	1	3
1959	10	7	1	..	1	1
1960	20	6	4	1	2	7
1961	8	3	..	1	..	4
				Gastro-Enteritis		
1957	508	298	116	2	14	78
1958	609	397	109	5	16	82
1959	497	292	103	7	5	90
1960	511	313	112	6	12	68
1961	534	375	83	3	12	61

Source: Registrar General
*Actually Age 0 (or children under 1 year)

TABLE 5. Notified Cases of Enteric Fever, 1954-1964

Year	Notified Cases
1954	667
1955	520
1956	499
1957	366
1958	422
1959	419
1960	574
1961	413
1962	309
1963	228
1964	289

Source: Chief Medical Officer

Appendix XV
Historical Note

In 1963, Guyana, which up until then had been a contributing territory to the regional University of the West Indies, established its own University, and in October of the same year, the first batch of 164 students was admitted. The new University began its operations in temporary premises loaned from Queen's College, the foremost Secondary School for boys, and of necessity teaching had to be carried out between 5 p.m. and 10 p.m.

The University of Guyana occupied its permanent site at Turkeyen, some five miles from the centre of Georgetown, in October 1969. The site of 140 acres was a gift from the Booker Group of Companies and the original ten buildings were made possible by capital grants from the Governments of the United Kingdom, Canada and Guyana.

At its inception the University offered only general Degree programmes confined to the Arts, Natural Sciences and Social Sciences. However, from 1966 Certificate and Diploma level programmes were introduced. The first Graduate programme was started in 1973.

The University currently has six faculties—Agriculture, Arts, Natural Sciences, Social Sciences, Education and Technology. The first students of the Faculty of Agriculture were admitted in 1977. The Faculty is still in the process of being established. Majors are offered in Agricultural Economics, Plant Science, Animal Science and Soil Science.

The Faculty of Arts began with major offerings in English, History, Geography, French, Mathematics and Spanish and later courses in Portuguese, Hindi, Dutch and Yoruba were added. A small Division of Creative Arts was established within the Faculty in 1975. The M.A. in Guyanese History, the first Graduate programme, was started in 1973.

Natural Sciences originally offered majors in Biology, Chemistry, Mathematics and Physics. In 1966, Diploma and Certificate programmes in Radiography and Medical Technology, respectively, were introduced. Of the former, only one batch of students was trained to meet the specific shortage of Radiographers at the time. Other batches were admitted in 1976 and 1977. A Diploma course in Pharmacy began in 1972. These Certificate and Diploma courses were administered by the Department of Biology until 1974 when a Department of Health Sciences was established. Its offerings now include the Diploma in Chemical Pathology and Microbiology, both introduced in 1977. M.Sc. degrees in Biology and Chemistry came into being in 1976 and 1977, respectively.

The original departments of the Faculty of Social Sciences were Economics and Business Administration, Government and Public Administration and Sociology. The Faculty was later reorganized and at present its departments are Economics, Management Studies, Political Science and Law, and Sociology. In 1975 an Institute of Development Studies was established within the Faculty. To its Degree programmes the Faculty added Diploma programmes in Public Administration (1966), Social Work (1971), Public Communication (1975), Accounting (1979), Personnel Management (1981), and by agreement, first-year teaching towards the LL.B. Degree of the University of the West Indies (1970). A Graduate programme in Economics began in 1977 and one in Political Science in 1978.

The Faculty of Education was established in 1967 and began its offerings with a postgraduate Diploma in Education. The Faculty increased its programmes with the introduction of a Certificate in Education (1972) and a Bachelor of Education (1975). In 1975 a Department of Extra Mural Studies was set up within the Faculty. A Master's Degree programme in Education was run in 1976/77.

In 1969 the Faculty of Technology was started. It offered a General Technical Diploma (GTD), and a Higher Technical Diploma (HTD) in Architecture and Building Technology, and in Civil, Electrical and Mechanical Engineering. To meet specific needs the Faculty has offered special one-year post HTD programmes in Public Health Engineering (1972), Highway Engineering (1975) and Architecture (1975). A Certificate and a Diploma course in Industrial Management were offered in 1972 and 1976, respectively. In 1977 the Faculty changed its existing TD and HTD programmes to Diploma in Technology and Bachelor of Engineering/Architecture programmes. An HTD in Mining Engineering began in 1979.

Full-time classes at the University were first introduced in 1969 in the Faculty of Technology. For the majority of the student population, that is the degree students in Arts, Natural and Social Sciences, full-time programmes became available in 1973.

From 1975 the University began accrediting programmes run by sister institutions in the Commonwealth Carribbean, e.g., Commonwealth Youth Programme; Commonwealth Regional Allied Health Programme and Health Science Tutors Programme.

However, the University must satisfy itself on matters relating to teaching, staff appointments, name of programme, admission requirements, regulations, course content, teaching methodology, examinations and examination procedures and also be represented on any governing or advisory board for any programme it is requested to certify.

The tuition fee of $100 per annum was abolished in 1974 and in 1975 participation in National Service was made a requirement for persons wishing to pursue programmes at the University.

Appendix XV   153

In 1980/81, the numbers of students registered were: Master's Degree, 20; Bachelor's Degrees, 1,356; Diplomas and Certificates, 625; Special students and Auditors, 133. The 1980 graduating class comprised 1 Master's and 235 Bachelor's Degrees, and 196 Diplomas and Certificates.[1]

---

[1] From the *University of Guyana Bulletin (1981–82)*, Publisher: University of Guyana, P.O. Box 10–1110, Georgetown, Guyana, pp. 8–9.

Notes

Chapter 1

1. Vere T. Daly, *A Short History of the Guyanese People* (British Guiana: Kitty Demerara, 1965), p. 15,
2. Raymond T. Smith, *British Guiana* (London: Oxford Univeristy Press, 1964), p. 16.
3. Daly, *A Short History* pp. 146-148.
4. Cheddi Jagan, *The West on Trial* (New York: International Publishers, 1966), p. 244.
5. *Ibid.* p. 402.
6. Harold A. Lutchman, "The Cooperative Republic of Guyana,"*Caribbean Studies*, 10,no.3 (1970):98.

Chapter 2

1. Material obtained from the administrator, Mr. Inder Persuad of Georgetown Hospital in August of 1964.
2. Material obtained from P. E. Fredericks, J. P. Barrister-at-law and former Director of the Guyana Sugar Producers' Association, 1966.
3. Material obtained from the British Guiana (Guyana) Development Program 1966-1977. Section VII—Health. (Georgetown: The Government Printery, 1977), pp. 1-12.

Chapter 3

1. Material obtained from P. E. Fredericks, J. P. Barrister at-law and former Director of the Guyana Sugar Producer's Association, 1966.

Chapter 4

1. Vere T. Daly, *A Short History of the Guyanese People* (British Guiana: Kitty Demerara, 1965), pp. 250-258.
2. *Ibid.*, pp. 266-269
3. Leo A. Despres, *Cultural Pluralism and Nationalistic Politics in British Guiana* (Chicago: Rand McNally Co., 1967), p. 51.
4. Report of a mission organized by the International Bank for Reconstruction and Development, *The Economic Development of British Guiana* (Georgetown: International Bank Printing, 1953), Introductions
5. *Sunday Chronicle* (Georgetown, Guyana: March 12, 1978), p. 8.
6. *Sunday Chronicle* (Georgetown, Guyana: March 26, 1978), p. 4.

7. *Sunday Chronicle* (Georgetown, Guyana: September 3, 1978), p. 7.
8. *Sunday Chronicle* (Georgetown, Guyana: March 18, 1979), p. 10
9. *Sunday Chronicle* (Georgetown, Guyana: October 15, 1978), p. 11
10. *Sunday Chronicle* (Georgetown, Guyana: August 12, 1979), p. 21.
11. Material obtained from P. E. Fredericks, J. P. Barrister-at-law and former Director of the Guyana Sugar Producers' Association, 1966. Permission to use this material was granted by the Director.

Chapter 5

1. Permission has been given by Dr. Patricia Rose to utilize this material on Hansen's Disease (Georgetown, 1979).

Chapter 6

1. M. H. Beaubrum, "Psychiatric Education for the Caribbean," *West Indian Medical Journal*, 15 (1966): 52.
2. Marcel A. Fredericks and Paul Mundy, "Social Backgrounds and Some Selected Attitudes of Physicians in a Developing Nation: Their Bearing on Medical Education for the Caribbean Area." *West Indian Medical* 16 (1967):216-221.
3. Permission to use material was obtained from P. E. Fredericks, formerly Director of the Guyana Sugar Producers' Association (Georgetown, 1966).
4. *Sunday Chronicle* (Georgetown, Guyana: June 25, 1978), p.6.
5. *Sunday Chronicle* (Georgetown, Guyana: March 5, 1978), p.11.

Chapter 7

1. *Sunday Chronicle* (Georgetown, Guyana: April 17, 1977), p. 7.
2. *Sunday Chronicle* (Georgetown, Guyana: February 18, 1979), p. 4.
3. *Sunday Chronicle* (Georgetown, Guyana: November 19, 1978), p. 18.
4. *Sunday Chronicle* (Georgetown, Guyana: February 13,1977), p. 11.
5. *Sunday Chronicle* (Georgetown, Guyana: November 12,1978), p. 6.
6. *Sunday Chronicle* (Georgetown, Guyana: February 13, 1977), p. 9.
7. *Sunday Chronicle* (Georgetown, Guyana: June 18, 1978), p. 4.
8. *Sunday Chronicle* (Georgetown, Guyana: July 23, 1978), p. 9.
9. *Sunday Chronicle* (Georgetown, Guyana: March, 1979), p. 9.
10. *Sunday Chronicle* (Georgetown, Guyana: August 5,1979), p. 18.
11. *Sunday Chronicle* (Gerogetown, Guyana: September 2, 1979), p. 3.

Chapter 8

1. T. Parsons "Definitions of health and illness in the light of American values and social structure." In E. G. Jaco, ed. *Patients, Physicians and Illness,2d ed., (New York: The Free Press, 1972). pp. 117-118.*

2. M. Zborowski, "*Cultural Components in Response to Pain*" *J Soc Issues* 8, no. 4 (1962): 16-30 See also his subsequent volume, *People in Pain* (San Francisco: Jossey-Bass, 1969).

3. W. J. Goode, *The Family* (Englewood Cliffs, N. J.: Prentice-hall, 1964) pp. 91-92.

4. H. B. Richardson, *Patients Have Families* (New York: The Commonwealth Fund, 1948), p. 76

5. T. K. Selkirk, "Hereditary Dark Teeth", *J. Pediatr* 46 (1955):192-199.

6. Pitirm A. Sorokin, *The Crisis of Our Age*, (New York: Dutton, 1942), p. 167

7. Goode, *The Family*, pp. 91-92.

8. R. J. Haggerty and J. J. Alpert "The Child, His Family, and Illness," *Postgrad Med J* 34 (1963):228-229.

9. *Ibid*.

10. J. J. Alpert, "The Functions of the Family Physician," *Conn. Med* 32(1975):664.

11. From Ministry of Health, Housing and Labour, Brickdam, Georgetown, Guyana, 1978.

Recommended Readings

Altick, Richard D. *The English Common Reader* (University of Chicago Press, 1957). An introductory study of the arts, crafts and customs of the Guiana Indians. 38th Annual Reports of the Bureau of American Ethnology, 1916-17. Washington, U. S. Government Printing Office, 1924. Additional studies of the arts, crafts and customs of the Guiana Indians, with special reference to those of Southern Guiana. Bureau Of American Ethnology Bulletin 91, Washington U. S. Government Printing Office, 1929.

Ayearst, Morley. *The British West Indies: The Search for Self-Government* (London: Allen and Unwin, 1960).

Beckett, J. Edgar. *From Hints on Agriculture in British Guiana: A Text Book for Use of the Small Farmer* (London: F. L. C., 1905).

Bhagwan, Moses. *Hitler's Force in Guiana* (Georgetown: New Guiana Co. Ltd. 1962).

Brett, W. H. *The Indian Tribes of Guiana* (London: Bell and Daldy, 1868). First published, New York, 1852.

Burnham, Forbes L. *The First Hundred Days of Consultative Democracy Under the People's National Congress—United States Government* (Georgetown, British Guiana: Lithographic Co. Ltd. 1965).

Cameron, N. E. *The Evolution of the Negro*, British Guiana Lithographic Co. Ltd., vol II. Book II (Georgetown: Guyana Argosy Co. Ltd., 1934).

Campbell, Sir Jock. "The Development and Organization of Bookers," paper delivered at the London School of Economics (London, November 1959).

Carew, Jan. *Black Midas* (London: Secker and Warburg, 1957).

Carter, Martin. *Poems of Resistance from British Guiana* (London: Lawrence and Wishart, 1954).

Chalmers, Robert (Baron). *The History of Currency in the British Colonies* (London: H. M. S. O., 1893).

Chase, Ashton. *122 Days Towards Freedom in Guiana* (Kitty, D. G., B's Printery, n.d.).

Clementi, Sir Cecil. *A Constitutional History of British Guiana* (London: MacMillan, 1937).

DeWeever, G. E. L. *The Children's Story of Guiana* (Georgetown: Argosy Ltd., n.d.).

Edun, Ayube M. *London's Heart-Probe and Britain's Destiny* (London: Arthur Stockwell, n.d.).

Gillin, John. *The Barama River Caribs of British Guiana*, papers of the Peabody Museum of Archaeology and Ethnology vol XIV, no. 2 (Cambridge, Mass: Harvard UNiversity Press, 1936).
Gravesande, Laurens Storm van's. *The Rise of British Guiana*, 2 vols. (London: Hakluyt Society, 1911).
Halperin, Ernst. *Racism and Communism in British Guiana* (Cambridge, Mass.: Massachusetts Institute of Technology Press 1964).
Harris, Wilson. *Palace of the Peacock* (London: Faber and Faber, 1961).
―――. *The Far Journey of Oudin* (London: Faber and Faber, 1961).
Hinden, Rita. *Local Government and the Colonies* A Report to the Fabian Colonial Bureau (London, 1950).
Hudson, W. H. *Green Mansions* (London: Duckworth 1904, reprinted 1947).
Im Thurn, E. F. *Among the Indians of Guiana* (London: Kegan Paul, Trench, 1883).
International Bank for Reconstruction and Development. *The Economic Development of British Guiana*, Report of a mission organized by the International Bank (Baltimore: Johns Hopkins Press, 1953).
Jagan, Chedd: *Fight for Freedom*. (Georgetown, Guyana: "National Printers" for Cheddi Jagan, c. 1953).
――― *Bitter Sugar* (Georgetown, Guyana: "National Printers" for Cheddi: Jagan, 1954).
―――. *Forbidden Freedom* (London: Lawrence and Wishart, 1954).
―――. *"Secret,"* Address to P.P.P. Congress on December 22, 1956 (duplicated only).
―――. *My Credo* (Georgetown, Guyana: New Guiana co Ltd., 1963).
―――*British Guiana's Future Peaceful or Violent?* (Georgetown: New Guiana Co. Ltd., 1964).
Jagan, Janet "Civil Liberties in British Guiana." *W.F.T.U. Bulletin*, March 1-15, 1953.
―――. *Election Facts* (Georgetown, Guyana: Magnet Printery, probably 1953).
―――. "Towards a Political Civil Service," *Thunder*, 14, no. 6 (1963).
Jayawardena, Chandra. *Conflict and Solidarity in a Guianese Plantation* (London: University of London Press, 1963).
King, Sidney, *Next Witness—An Appeal to World Opinion* (Georgetown: Labour Advocate Job Printing Department, July 1962).
Kirke, Henry. *Twenty-five Years in British Guiana* (London, 1898). (Georgetown: Guiana Edition, No. 12, 1948.)
London Missionary Society (The). *Report of the Proceedings Against the Late Rev. J. Smith of Demerara* (London 1824).
Mahraj, Deoroop. *Election Manifesto for 1953* (unknown).
Mittelholzer, E. A. *Corentyne Thunder* (London: Eyre and Spottiswode, 1941).
―――. *Shadows Move Among Them* (London: Peter Nevil, 1951).
―――. *Children of Kaywana* (London: Peter Nevil, 1952).

———. *Life and Death of Sylvia* (London: Secker and Warburg, 1953).
———. *The Harrowing of Hubertus* (London: Secker and Warburg, 1954).
———. *My Bones and My Flute* (London: Secker and Warburg, 1955).
Nath, Dwarka. *A History of the Indians in British Guiana* (London: Nelson, 1950).
Nueman, Peter. *British Guiana* (London: Oxford University Press, 1964).
———. "Racial Tension in British Guiana," *Race*, May 1962.
Pinckard, Dr. George. *Letters from Guiana* (1796-1797) Georgetown, Guyana: Daily Chronicle Press, 1937-1938).
Ragatz, L. J. *The Fall of the Planter Class in the British Caribbean 1763-1833* (London: Oxford University Press, 1928)
Raleigh, Sir Walter. *The Discovery of the Large and Beautiful Empire of Guiana*, reprinted from edition of 1596, ed. by Sir H. Schomburgk (London: Hakluyt Society, 1848). (Hakluyt Society No. 3).
Reno, Philip. *The Ordeal of British Guiana* (New York: Monthly Review Press, 1964).
Rodway, J. *Guiana: British, Dutch and French* (London: Unwin, 1912)
———. *History of British Guiana from 1668* (Georgetown: Argosy, 1891).
———. *The Story of Georgetown* (Georgetown: Argosy Co. 1920).
Roth W. E. An Inquiry into the Animism and Folklore of the Guiana Indians. 30th Annual Report of the Bureau of American Ethnology, 1908-09. (Washington: U.S. Government Printing Office, 1915).
Rubin, Vera, ed. *Caribbean Studies: A Symposium* (Jamaica: Institute of Social and Economic Research, University College of the West Indies, 1957).
Schomburgk, Robert. *A Description of British Guiana, 1840-44* (London: Simpkin, Marshall, 1840). (Guiana edition, No 17, Georgetown, 1922.)
Smith, Raymond T. *British Guiana* (London: Oxford University Press, 1962).
———. *The Negro Family in British Guiana* (London: Routledge and Kegan Paul, 1956).
Smith, Raymond T. "Some Social Characteristics of Indian Immigrants to British Guiana," *Population Studies*. 12, no. 1 (1959).
Steward, J. H., ed. *Handbook of South American Indians* (Washington, D.C. : U.S. Government Printing Office, 1948). Smithsonian Institute Bureau of American Ethnology Bulletin 143. Vol. 3: The Tropical Forest Tribes, Parts 5 and 6.
Swan, Michael. *British Guiana: The Land of the Six Peoples* (London: H.M.S.O., 1957).
Waterton, Charles. *Wanderings in South America* (London: MacMillan, 1878).
Webber, A.R.F. *Centenary History and Handbook of British Guiana* (Georgetown: Argosy Co. Ltd., 1931).
Williams, Eric. *The Negro in the Caribbean* (Manchester: Panaf Service, 1944).

———. *Capitalism and Slavery* (Chapel Hill: University of North Carolina Press, 1944).

Young, Allan. *The Approaches to Local Self-Government in British Guiana* (London: Longmans, 1958).

Young, M. and Willmott, P. *Family and Kinship in East London* (London: Routledge and Kegan Paul, 1957).

Glossary

Acchar. Hot condiment.
Amerindian. (American Indian). Population is comprised of nine tribal groupings throughout the ninety major Amerindian villages to be found in Guyana. The Groups are Carib, Arawak, Wai-Wai, Akawaio, Makushi, Warrau, Wapishiana, Arecuna and Patamona. There are also dialects peculiar to the individual groups which are spoken but not written; a few are common to the various groups.
Amuku. A lake situated west of the Rupununi River.
Apple. Small and sweet fruit when ripe.
Awara. Small fruit. It has a fibrous flesh which encases a huge central seed. Possesses very little flavor.
Baccoo. Folk figure which represents a tiny man who is kept in a bottle and is fed on bananas and milk. He brings his owner jewels and gold. Unaccountable wealth is frequently attributed to ownership of a Baccoo.
Baigan Choka. Consists of eggplant prepared with garlic and roasted. The skin is then peeled, and the residue is mixed with onion, salt, and heated oil. There are other forms of choka prepared from salted cod, coconut, tomatoes, smoked herring, and potatoes.
Baiganie. Sliced eggplant dipped in a mixture of ground split peas and condiments, then fried.
Bake. A form of bread, somewhat similar to roti, which is fried in oil.
Bananas. Five distinct types grow in Guyana.
Bara. Ground split peas mixed with condiments, similar to Phulouri.
Barima River. Has the following tributaries: the Aruku, Kaituma, Anabisi, Whanamaparu, and Whenna.
Bhaji. Spinach.
Bird Pepper. The hottest type of pepper, small and thin. Main ingredient in the local hot pepper sauce.
Black Pudding. A sausage made of boiled rice and various meats.
Bora. Dark-green vegetables about twelve to eighteen inches in length.
Boulanger. Vegetable also called "eggplant."
Breadfruit. Large, round fruit which is used as a vegetable.
Breadnut. Short, dull, regular spikes cover the skin of this round yellow-

green fruit. The white nuts are surrounded in a white pulp. The nuts are eaten after being boiled.
Buck. Somewhat similar to the apple in size, shape and flavor.
Burnham, Linden F. S. Formerly the Prime Minister of Guyana. At present, he is the President of the Republic.
Bush Dai-Dai. Folk figure that is seen in gold-rich jungle areas and is often the pork-knocker's ruin. Men have been reported greying overnight or being driven mad following an encounter with such a folk figure.
Calaloo. Vegetable grown in several varieties. Sometimes used as spinach.
Canje River. A tributary of the Berbice River.
Cashew. Small, kidney-shaped nut. It has a good flavor and may be eaten raw.
Cassareep. Liquid extracted from bitter cassava.
Cassava. A staple food of the Amerindian population which is used in a variety of forms such as cassava bread, cassareep, farine (cereal), and cassiri (wine).
Cayenne. Long and slim pepper resembling a plantain except slightly shorter.
Chana. Also called split peas in North America. The raw chana is soaked overnight, fried in deep oil and then sprinkled with salt.
Che Che Ra. A vegetable in the form of squash. It is long and slim. Sometimes used in curry.
Chives. See shallots.
Chow Chow. Unripe mangoes sprinkled with pepper, salt, and vinegar.
Chung, Arthur. Former President of the Cooperative Republic of Guyana.
Chutney. Sweet or hot condiment.
Coastal Plain. The White Sand Region terminates a short distance from the coast-line in a series of hills about 100 feet high. Between these hills and the sea there is a coastal plain of varying widths which has been formed by recent accretion. Much of this area is below the level of high tides and is protected from inundation by various forms of sea defenses.
Cocrite. Small oval fruit with a firm, brown skin. The beige pulp encases a huge seed.
Cook-Up Food. A local term used to describe various foods which are cooked together. For example, meats, fish, rice, lentils, and vegetables are all cooked in the same utensil.
Coolie Jumbie. Appears suddenly in the area of a burial ground or a sugar factory. The dhoti-clad figure seems to reflect the freed slaves' anxiety at the appearance of a newly arrived indentured laborer.

Coraila. Vegetable resembling a cucumber with pointed ends. It is sometimes fried with salted cod fish.
Curry. Meat or vegetables cooked with special condiments such as curry powder, tumeric, and cumin seeds.
Custard Apple. Green fruit approximately the size of a large orange. It has a sweet, moist, cream-colored pulp which is mustard-like in flavor.
Dasheen. Large brown vegetable covered with roots. Used mainly in soups and stews.
Demerara River. Has the following tributaries: the Kamuni, Kuliserabo, Madeqini, Moblissa, and the Kara-Kara.
Dholl. Boiled split peas somewhat similar to split pea soup with condiments added.
Dholl Poorie. Roti filled with boiled split peas.
Diwali or Deepavali. The Hindu festival of lights, characterized by the illumination of Diyas (small earthenware lamps) in homes, electric lights in shops and in public buildings, and fireworks. It is a time of joy, revelry and good fellowship.
Dunk. Apple-shaped fruit, It is used as a substitute for prunes.
Dye. Known as tumeric or saffron. Form of spice which gives a coloring to foods such as curried chicken.
Eddoe. Dark brown root vegetable. Used in soups and stews.
Essequibo River. Has the following tributaries: the Mazaruni, Cuyuni, Potaro, Siparuni, Rupununi, and Kiyuwini.
Five Fingers. Smooth-skinned fruit with five length-wise ridges so that if it is sliced across, each slice is shaped like a star.
Foo-Foo. The term given to plantains when they are boiled and curshed in a wooden block (sometimes called a "mata") by a very heavy piece of wood (sometimes called a "mata stick").
Garlic Pork. A delicacy usually prepared during the Christmas holidays. It is a traditional Portuguese food in which pork is preserved in garlic and thyme. Pork and other ingredients are placed in a jar and carefully sealed. Pieces of meat are removed with a very clean fork from the jar, and these are carefully fried and used for breakfast.
Genip. Small fruit with a thick, rough, green skin and an apricot-colored flesh which encloses one large stone or pit.
Georgetown. The capital of Guyana; it is situated at the mouth of the Demerara River on the eastern bank. It is the main harbor, the seat of government, and the chief commercial center. It has an estimated population of 183,000.
Ghee. Clarified butter used in cooking. It is a necessity in Hindu religious ceremonies.
Gigioli, Dr. George. Was a retired medical advisor to the Sugar Pro-

ducers' Association. He laid the basic foundations for the eradication of malaria by means of a very skillfully designed scheme of house spraying with DDT.

Golden Apple. Resembles a North American apple in consistency. It is about three inches long and oval in shape. It is generally eaten raw or made into juice, jelly or sauce.

Gooseberry. Tiny, round, smooth-skinned berry. Has a white pulp and a single seed. Eaten with salt or made into jelly, pies, or tarts.

Gos. Meat.

Greenheart. A very sturdy timber used to build houses.

Grenadilla. Oval, medium-sized fruit with a white pulp. It grows on a vine and is eaten fresh or used for making juice or ice cream.

Guava. Small, yellow fruit with many tiny seeds. It may be eaten raw, stewed, or made into juice, jelly, or "guava cheese".

Gulgula. A flour dumpling filled with a sweet coconut mixture.

Guyana. Lies on the northeast of their continent of South America, bordering Venezuela, Brazil and Surinam between latitudes 1^0 North and 9^0 North, and longitudes 56^0 west and 62^0 West. Its total area is estimated at 83,000 square miles. Approximately 85 per cent of the area is forested and 10.5 per-cent is savannah country; the remainder is of flat alluvial clays. The country has a seacoast of roughly 270 miles, extending from near the mouth of the Orinoco River on the west to the Coventyne River on the east and may be divided into five major physiographic areas: the Kanuku Mountains, the Pakaraima Mountains, the Savannah Mountains, the White Sand Region and the Coastal Plain.

Jack Fruit. Fruit about sixteen or more inches in length and at least eight inches in diameter. The covering skin is made up of dull green spikes. The inside contains large black seeds surrounded by a white pulp which is eaten.

Jagan, Dr. Cheddi. Leader of the opposition party (PPP). He held the position of General Secretary of the party.

Jan Sin Yu. Steamed fish with mixed vegetable dressing.

Jilebi. Fried yeast mixture. It includes flour, sugar, spices, yeast, and syrup. Form of sweet meat.

Kaieteur Fall. Was discovered on April 29, 1870, by Charles Barrington Brown. It is situated on the Potaro River, a tributary of the Essequibo River. The water of Kaieteru Fall flows over a sandstone conglomerate tableland into a deep valley—a drop of 741 feet or five times the height of Niagara Falls.

Kanaima. Folk figure that inflicts sickness, vengeance and even death. It functions through an animal, a person, or an inanimate object.

Kanuku Mountains. A broad belt of rugged country with numerous peaks rising to about 2,500 feet above sea level. Extends roughly east-west across the southern part of the country. The hills are almost completely forest-covered and consist mainly of metamorphic rocks.

Kasheerie. Prepared from cassava which for centuries provided the staple diet of the Amerindians. (See Cassava.) Kasheerie is prepared by chewing the cassava granules and then placing the residue in a large drum. Water is then added, and the cassava brew is allowed to ferment for one week. Color is then added to the brew by the use of grated potatoes.

Kuru Kuru Cooperative College. Located about 35 miles south of Georgetown. It was incorporated in 1973, and its affairs are managed by a Board of Governors.

Kyk-over-al. An island situated off Kartabu, at the confluence of the Cuyuni, Mazaruni, and Essequibo Rivers. From this position, a magnificent view over the Guyuni, Mazaruni, and Essequibo Rivers is presented, hence the name which means "See Over All."

Leguan. An island of about eighteen square miles. Situated west of the Demerara River.

Leprosy. The name given in Biblical times to various cutaneous diseases, especially those of a chronic or contagious nature; it probably embraces psoriasis and leukoderma. (Also called Hansen's disease.)

Lime. Fruit about the size of a ping-pong ball. Somewhat similar to the lemon in taste.

Linden. A town located on the Demerara River approximately 67 miles from Georgetown. It includes the town formerly known as Mackenzie, site of the operations of the Guyana Mining Enterprises, and the two villages of Wismar and Christianburg. The area of the town is approximately 55 square miles.

Machhali Ka Talkari. Stewed fish.

Mamey Apple. Fruit about the size of a small grapefruit. Eaten raw or stewed.

Masacurraman. Folk figure which represents a snake haired giant. It rises out of the water to devour the observer.

Mashramani. An Amerindian celebration. It means "celebration after cooperative effort." This celebration has been infused into the culture, and it is now the biggest and most colorful national affair touching the State's 5,000 communities.

Massala. Curry Paste. Ingredients are ground on a stone. The paste includes onion, garlic, and red pepper.

Mauby Bark. Has a bitter flavoring for a popular local drink called mauby.

168   Glossary

Metemgee.   An African dish made with yam, plantain, and cassava. Meat and fish are sometimes included. It is prepared by using coconut milk rather than water in boiling the food.

Mittai,   sweetmeat which is made of dough, fried in oil and dipped in syrup.

Mohan Bhog.   Form of sweet cake. Includes flour, soda, spice, sugar, raisins, milk, and ghee.

Moon-Gazer.   Folk figure which represents a male with formless legs. He stands at corssroads looking up at the moon. If his legs are touched, it is believed that the skin will grow.

Mora.   A lumber utilized to erect houses and construct furniture.

Murgi Talkari.   Curried chicken.

New Amsterdam.   An old Dutch town which is situated on the eastern bank of Berbice River. It has an estimated population of 20,000.

Ng Heung Ja Gai.   Fried spiced chicken.

Ochro.   Same as okra. A slender vegetable with soft seeds and a slimy substance.

Ol Higue.   A folk figure that travels as a ball of fire settling on a tree or a lamp post outside the intended victim's house. In this form the hag enters the house through the key hole. Once inside, she attacks young children, sucking their blood through punctures she makes in their necks. A stiff neck is often taken as evidence that Ol Higue has paid a visit. The child might become seriously ill or even die.

Otaheite Apple.   Small pear-shaped fruit. It is used for making jelly and jams.

Pakaraima Mountains.   Form a broad belt of mountainous areas which extend east-southeast across the northern half of the country from its frontier with Venezuela and Brazil to the Berbice River. The Pakaraimas consist mainly of a series of sandstone plateaus of varying altitudes and terminate northeastward in a long, irregular escarpment 1,000 to 3,000 feet high, which runs roughly parallel to, and 140 miles distant from, the coastline.

Pak Choy.   Green vegetable used in Chinese cooking. Can be a substitute for chopped celery.

Paratha.   Roti with ghee-flour, soda, and slat are mixed. The dough is rolled and cooked on a hot baking stone.

Pawpaw (Papaya).   Fruit served with lemon juice or in a fruit cup. Green pawpaws may be cooked as a vegetable or treated as a green apple.

Peda.   A sweetmeat which is similar to fudge.

Pepperpot.   Made of cassareep, pork and beef, and pepper. It is a national dish of Guyana, eaten by all cultural groups in the society.

Phagwah.   A joyous Hindu festival celebrating the triumph of good over evil.

Phulouri. Ground split peas mixed with water, flour, salt and massala.
Pine. Word used for pineapple.
Plantain. A kind of tropical plant which is related to the banana. Its fruit, which resembles the banana, is consumed after it is boiled. At times it is crushed and eaten with soups and meats.
PNC. The Peoples' National Congress Party which is now the ruling party.
Polowrie. Consists of ground split peas mixed with condiments.
Pomegranate. Fruit about the size of an orange. It has many small seeds in a pink pulp.
Pork-knocker. Seeker of gold and diamonds.
Psidium. Fruit about the size of a large plum. The pulp encases five flat seeds. It is used to make jelly.
Puri. Made of dough somewhat similar to roti, but it is deep fried in ghee.
Sapodilla. Brown-skinned fruit about the size of a large plum. The pulp has several large flat black seeds in the center. It is served in fruit salad, punch, and ice cream.
Savannah Mountains. Consist mainly of volcanic rocks. Situated south of a line joining the Echilebar and Separuni rivers.
Seaside Grape. Fruit resembling a cherry.
Semitoo. Fruit about the size of a lemon. Has a thin layer of pulp which surrounds a large number of black seeds enclosed in a juice-filled skin. Used in fruit salads and in local rum punch.
Sey Foo Gnar Choy. Bean sprouts with tomatoes.
Shallots (Chives). Member of the onion family. It has a garlicky flavor. Used as a substitute for onions.
Sorrell. A seasonal fruit available only at Christmas. Used to make juice, jelly or liqueur.
Sour Fig. A very small banana. It is yellow when ripe.
Sourie. Cucumber-shaped fruit about two inches long. Sometimes eaten with salt or used to make a cold drink.
Soursop. Large green-skinned fruit covered in soft spines. Black tiny seeds are surrounded by pulp. Sometimes used in ice cream.
Star Anise. Star-shaped brown seed which is used mainly in Chinese cooking.
Star Apple. Purple fruit. Used for desserts or jams.
Sugar Apple. Fruit about the size of a tangerine. Resembles a pine cone. Sometimes used for making ice cream.
Sweet Fig. A rather tiny banana about two inches long and similar to sour fig in appearance.
Tamarind. Elongated, flat pod containing black seeds. May be eaten raw, but it is usually dried and used as a condiment in various dishes.

Tangelo. Large citrus fruit resembling a tangerine.
Tannia. Root vegetable. Exterior is covered with roots. Used in soups and stews.
Tapakuma. A lake situated southwest of Anna Regina.
Univeristy of Guyana. Established by ordinance in April, 1963.
Vanilla Essence. From "Vanilla" pods which are soaked in rum. Used in flavoring various sweet dishes.
White Lady. Folk figure that represents the wife of an estate manager in the colonial period. She supposedly lures children to their deaths.
White Sand Region. Formed mainly of stratified sands and clays which were deposited in the sea or in the broad estuaries or deltas of rivers. Recent elevation of the region has led to erosion and partial removal of these deposits by the large rivers.
Whytee. Yellow-green pod which has several black seeds with a white substance.
Wiri Wiri Pepper. Tiny red pepper, comparatively mild.
Yam. Root vegetable. It is shaped like a potato with several protrusions.
Yaws. An infectious disease of the tropics, marked by febrile disturbances, rheumatic pains, and an eruption of aggregated rounded or flattened turbercles capped with a caseous (cheese-like) crust.
You-man-nabi. The birthday of Mohammed, the prophet of Islam.

Special thanks are extended to Mrs. Anna Broomes for her valued assistance in dealing with foods and beverages in this glossary.

Index

(This index focuses on significant discussions of important topics)

Administrative districts,
  Health facilities, 141-146
Adult education, 135, *see also*
  Education, Schools
Africa, 5, 111
Alleluiah religion, 115
Amerindians, 102, 103, 106, 109-111, 113-116
Area, 1, 101
"Bartica Triangle", 102
Bauxite, 102, 137
Birth rates, 96-98, 147-150
"Bush doctor", 80
Caribbean, 104
Cassava, 114
Children and health care, 40
Chinese, 4, 121
Christian, 10, 106, 115, 125-126
Cities and towns, 105-106
Climate, 103-104
Coastal plain, 102
Community aid in health services development, 23
Constitution, 117, 119
Creolese, 106
Culture, 3-7, 114, 121-123
DDT, 34-36, 54-55
Death rates, 96-98, 147-150
Denbow, Enid, Dr., 75
Dental care, 84-85
Diamond fields, 103

District Hospitals, 20-21
Drainage, 102
Drug abuse, 92-93
Drugs, 39, 62-63
Dutch colonial era, 104, 106, 109
Education, 43-50, 56, 131-135,
  see also Schools
Emancipation Act, 56
English, 3, 10, 46, 106
Environmental cleanliness, 37
Environmental Sanitation Program, 18
Family
  Problems, 87-88
  Sick role, 88-91
  Typology, 91-92
  Stress, 92
Fertility rates, 99
Festivals, religious, 125-126
Filaria, 17-18
Flag, Guyana, 127
Folk medicine, 79-86
Food, 4-5, 139
Food adulteration, 93
Georgetown, 2, 40, 51, 76, 81, 105, 106
Georgetown Hospital, 11-12, 21-22, 75, 93, 95
Geriatric Unit, 23
Giglioli, George, Dr., 51-56, 67, 70-75

Gold, 103
Government, 2, 7-10, 41, 50, 119
Hansen's Disease, 22, 57-65
   Cure, 57-58
Health care,
   Changes, 87-100
   Facilities, 94-96, 141-146
   Death/Birth Rates, 96-98, 147-150
   Fertility Rates, 99
Health care development: 1933-1966, 12-16
Health education, 41
   History, 43-46
   Current, 46-50, 82-84
   Giglioli, 51-56
Health services development, 24-25
Health services structure, 17, *see also* Public Health Services
Herb cures, Indigenous, 38-40
Highland region, 103
Hilly sand and clay area, 102
Hindu, 4, 5, 106, 121, 125-126
Hinterland Services, 23, 113
History (Guyana), 109-111
Hookworn, 74
Illness, 7
Industries, 137
Infant mortality rates, 147-150
Infection transmission, Hansen's Disease, 59-65
Islands, 104
Lakes, 104
Language, 106
Leprosy, *see* Hansen's Disease
Maize, 103
Malaria, 17, 73-74
   Eradication campaign, 28-37
Manganese, 103
Maternal and Child Welfare Clinics, 18

Medical research, 51-56
Mental health, 93
Mental illness, 80, 93
Miller, Carlyle, Dr., 75
Missionaries, 114
Mountains, 103
Muslim, 4, 106, 121, 125-126
Parasitic infestation, 18
Physicians,
   Role of, 67
   Social backgrounds, 67-68
   Attitudes toward medical profession, 68-69, 76-77
   Outstanding, 70-76
Political situation, *see* Government
Population, 1, 3, 101, 113
Ports, 107
Portugese, 3, 10, 111
Preventive medicine, 17, 19
Primary schools, 131-132, *see also* Education, Schools
Public health services, 27-41
   Before independence, 27-28
   Current, 37-40
Religion, 106, 125-126
Resources, 2
Rice, 102, 137
Rivers, 1-2, 103, 105
Rose, Patricia, Dr., 57-65
Savannahs, 103
Schools, 46-49, 53, 114, 131-136, *see also* Education
Sea defense, 102
Secondary schools, 132-133, *see also* Education, Schools
Snake bites, 80
South America, 101
Special education, 135, *see also* Education, Schools
Sugar, 102, 137

Teacher education, 134-135, *see also* Education, Schools
Timber, 102
Time, local, 101
Tobacco, 103
Tuberculosis, 22, 40
    Pulmonary, 18
Typhoid, 19
U.S. AID, 39, 40
United States of America, 97-99
University of Ghana, 49, 135, 151-153, *see also* Education, Schools
Urdu, 106
Vocational schools, 134, *see also* Education, Schools
Voodoo, 85
Warpeha, Raymond, L., Dr., 75-76
Weddings, 5-6

DATE DUE

GAYLORD · PRINTED IN U.S.A.